Innovations in WASH Impact Measures

DIRECTIONS IN DEVELOPMENT
Infrastructure

Innovations in WASH Impact Measures

Water and Sanitation Measurement Technologies and Practices to Inform the Sustainable Development Goals

Evan Thomas, Luis Alberto Andrés, Christian Borja-Vega, and German Sturzenegger, Editors

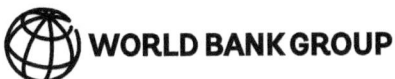

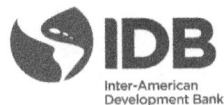

WORLD BANK GROUP

IDB
Inter-American
Development Bank

Contents

Box

Figures

Photos

Tables

Foreword

Achieving the ambitious targets of the Sustainable Development Goals (SDGs) will require new approaches, tools, and technologies. The beginning of 2018 marks 1,000 days since the SDGs were gaveled into existence in New York, meaning the SDG era is well underway. SDG 6 commits to "ensure availability and sustainable management of water and sanitation for all," which is an opportunity for the sector as well as a challenge for those tasked with measuring and reporting progress.

Until recently, countries reported on their populations' access to water and sanitation by distinguishing between "improved" and "unimproved" coverage. Despite the impressive progress during the Millennium Development Goals (MDGs) era, in 2015, 660 million people were drinking from unimproved sources such as unprotected dug wells, and 2.4 billion lacked improved sanitation facilities.

SDG 6 commits to universal access to water, sanitation, and hygiene (WASH) under a new, broader, and more refined monitoring framework. The binary unimproved/improved distinction is replaced by the concept of "safely managed" services. For water (target 6.1), it requires that the household's drinking water source be on premises and that water be available when needed and free of fecal and locally relevant chemical contamination. For sanitation (target 6.2), emphasis is placed on the links in the sanitation chain from initial defecation through waste management (including containment, disposal, and transport of human excreta), and on the availability of an appropriate handwashing facility. Monitoring these components and inequalities will help to measure progress toward the longer-term aim of universal access.

The WASH sector is complex, and the questions we seek to answer and the indicators we seek to track are equally complex. *Innovations in WASH Impact Measures* presents insightful, clearly explained, and practical approaches, tools, and technologies for those working in monitoring and evaluation. The book reviews the landscape of proven and emerging technologies, methods, and approaches that can support the measurement of the complex WASH indicators proposed for targets 6.1 and 6.2. It provides a comprehensive review of topics from big data to behavior change, satellites to safe sanitation, and presents these issues in an accessible and applicable way.

Much of its content relates to technology and its potential to transform the way we collect and analyze data. One example is that of satellite-based remote sensing, which can assist with the accounting of water use and productivity. These data facilitate efficient management of water resources on a large scale. Using remotely sensed data and having access to more frequent and more comprehensive information can lead to better decision making. For example, the book reveals that sensor technology combined with video images is an effective and unobtrusive way of observing and recording handwashing behavior. Sensors can help measure sanitation interventions in other ways too—such as how an ordinary looking bar of soap with embedded technology can provide accurate estimates of how regularly people wash their hands after defecating.

As more information is generated and new technologies are used, more possibilities for analysis are created. Monitoring can happen in real time, allowing adjustments to be made as soon as they're needed. This book helps discover trends that were previously hiding in plain sight. And it improves our accountability to the people we serve, because it allows us to provide new kinds of robust evidence of impact.

This book also identifies some of the shortcomings of traditional monitoring and evaluation methods. While household surveys and censuses still have a role to play, they can be most useful when integrated with other sources such as water quality testing and earth observations. The book does not recommend one technology above another. Their application should always be context-specific.

Effective monitoring is needed to ensure interventions are having the impact we hope for or to adjust them in a timely manner. Practitioners will find in these pages a wealth of information and inspiration to ensure just that. Monitoring progress is a journey, not a destination, and our institutions are traveling together on this ongoing journey. Our hope is that, by making this information publicly available, we will inspire you and other WASH practitioners to begin using these technologies when monitoring SDG6, so this ambitious goal is more likely to be achieved.

Guangzhe Chen   José Agustín Aguerre
Senior Director   *Manager*
Water Global Practice   *Infrastructure and Energy Sector*
The World Bank Group   *The Inter-American Development Bank*

Acknowledgments

Innovations in WASH Impact Measures: Water and Sanitation Measurement Technologies and Practices to Inform the Sustainable Development Goals was edited by Evan Thomas (Oregon Health and Science University, Portland State University), Luis Alberto Andrés (The World Bank), Christian Borja-Vega (The World Bank), and Germán Sturzenegger (The Inter-American Development Bank). The publication includes contributions from Christina Barstow (University of Colorado at Boulder), Kwasi Boateng (Portland State University), Thomas Clasen (Emory University), Katie Fankhauser (Oregon Health and Science University), Libbet Loughnan (World Bank), Tom Slaymaker (United Nations Children's Fund/World Health Organization Joint Monitoring Programme), and Nick Turman-Bryant (Portland State University).

The team also values the ongoing support and technical inputs from Stefan Buss, Fabiana Velasques de Paula Machado, Gastón Gertner, and Raúl Munoz Castillo from the Inter-American Development Bank, and from Richard Damania, Antonio Rodriguez Serrano, Aleix Serrat Capdevila, Avjeet Singh, Maria Angelica Sotomayor, and Malar Veerappan from the World Bank.

The findings, interpretations, and conclusions expressed in this document are those of the authors and do not necessarily reflect the views of the executive directors of the World Bank or the Inter-American Development Bank, the governments they represent, or the counterparts consulted or engaged with during the study process. Any factual errors are, as well, the responsibility of the editors.

About the Editors and Contributors

Editors

Evan Thomas, PhD, PE, MPH is an Associate Professor of Mechanical Engineering at Portland State University and of Public Health at the Oregon Health and Science University, Portland State University School of Public Health. Evan holds a PhD in aerospace engineering sciences from the University of Colorado at Boulder, is a registered Professional Engineer (P.E.) in environmental engineering, and holds a masters in public health from the Oregon Health and Science University. Evan is also the founder and Chief Executive Officer of SweetSense Inc., an "Internet of Things" technology start-up focused on emerging markets.

Luis Alberto Andrés is Lead Economist in the Water Global Practice at the World Bank. Earlier, Dr. Andrés held positions in the Sustainable Development Department for the Latin America and Caribbean and the South Asia regions. His work at the World Bank involves both analytical and advisory services, with a focus on infrastructure, mainly in water and energy sectors, impact evaluations, private sector participation, regulation, and empirical microeconomics. He worked with numerous Latin American, South Asian, and East European governments. Before joining the World Bank, he was the Chief of Staff for the Secretary of Fiscal and Social Equity for the Government of Argentina and held other positions in the Chief of the Cabinet of Ministers and the Ministry of Economy. He holds a PhD in economics from the University of Chicago and has authored books, chapters, monographs, and articles on development policy issues.

Christian Borja-Vega is an Economist in the Water Global Practice at the World Bank, with 10 years of experience in development organizations. His experience with the World Bank focuses on water sector operations and economic analysis. He also was sector program coordinator of the Strategic Impact Evaluation Fund (SIEF) where he managed Water Supply, Sanitation, and Hygiene (WASH) Impact Evaluations in Africa, Latin America and the Caribbean, and East Asia regions. Prior to working in the World Bank, he held positions as research analyst at the Social Development Secretariat in Mexico and the Mexican Health Foundation. Christian has co-authored several publications in academic and policy journals, as well as in specialized magazines and newspapers. He earned a BA in economics at ITESM in Mexico and a masters in public policy at the University of Chicago, and he is a PhD candidate in civil engineering at the University of Leeds in the United Kingdom.

Germán Sturzenegger is a Water and Sanitation Senior Specialist at the Inter-American Development Bank (IDB). He has participated in the design and implementation of water and sanitation projects throughout Latin America and the Caribbean. Germán leads the impact evaluation and behavior change agendas, supporting the development of empirical evidence in the WASH sector. He also leads the recycling and green infrastructure agendas at IDB's Water and Sanitation Division, where he works on advancing watershed conservation and inclusive recycling projects throughout the region. Germán has authored several publications on sustainability, fostering water and sanitation markets, and the challenges the sector faces under the new development agenda. He is a Fulbright Scholar, holds a master's degree in public policy from Harvard University, and has been actively involved in the development world for more than 10 years.

Contributors

Christina Barstow currently serves as Water Evaluation and Behavior Change Advisor within the American Association for the Advancement of Science Fellowship. Christina's work has focused primarily on large-scale program implementation and research in the water and energy sectors. Christina holds a PhD in environmental engineering from the University of Colorado at Boulder.

Kwasi Boateng earned his BSc in civil engineering from the University of Science and Technology, Ghana, and his MS in engineering technology management from Western Kentucky University. He worked as a research assistant at Portland State University, where his focus was on experimental design and data analysis. He is currently an energy analyst for JouleSmart Solutions, a smart building management firm in the Portland, Oregon, area.

Thomas Clasen, an epidemiologist, is Professor of Environmental Health and Rose Salamone Gangarosa Chair of Sanitation and Safe Water at the Rollins School of Public Health, Emory University, where he teaches courses on the critical appraisal of water, sanitation, and hygiene research and on environmental health policy. He has led more than $40 million in research on household-level environmental health interventions in low-income countries. His work has been published in leading journals, including *The Lancet Global Health*, *The BMJ*, *PLOS Medicine*, *Environmental Health Perspectives*, *WHO Bulletin*, *Epidemiology*, and the *International Journal of Epidemiology*. Professor Clasen is the chief advisor to the World Health Organization in developing the first set of *Guidelines for Sanitation and Health*. He holds an MSc (control of infectious diseases) and

PhD from the University of London; he also holds a JD from Georgetown University Law Center.

Katie Fankhauser has been involved professionally and academically in the implementation and analysis of energy, water, and sanitation projects in East Africa for several years. She holds a master's in public health in biostatistics from the Oregon Health and Science University, Portland State University School of Public Health. Katie has worked as a program manager for DelAgua Health in Rwanda and SweetSense Inc. She is a 2015 EPA STAR Fellow, and her research includes environmental impact assessments in Rwanda and Oregon.

Libbet Loughnan is a water, sanitation, hygiene, and statistics and monitoring specialist. She consults as an adviser to the World Bank Water Global Practice and country teams on the international WASH indicators. Formerly, she was with the World Health Organization/United Nations Children's Fund Joint Monitoring Programme for Water Supply, Sanitation, and Hygiene (WHO/UNICEF JMP) and the Data and Analytics Section/Division of Data, Research, and Policy in UNICEF headquarters. She also worked as the director of a children's health and development foundation in China.

Tom Slaymaker is a Senior Statistics and Monitoring Specialist (WASH) in the Division of Data, Research, and Policy at UNICEF Headquarters in New York. He has nearly 20 years' experience working on water and sanitation, mainly in Africa and Asia, and currently manages the WHO/UNICEF Joint Monitoring Programme for Water Supply, Sanitation, and Hygiene.

Nick Turman-Bryant is a PhD candidate in systems science at Portland State University. Nick uses statistical tools to derive actionable insights from sensors that are installed on cookstoves, latrines, borehole pumps, and hand pumps in Ethiopia, Kenya, and Rwanda. Nick also holds a master's in energy, technology, and policy from Humboldt State University, where he worked with the Schatz Energy Research Center.

Abbreviations

CFU	colony forming units
DHS	Demographic and Health Surveys
E. coli	*Escherichia coli*
EPA	U.S. Environmental Protection Agency
FEWS NET	Famine Early Warning System Network
GPS	Global Positioning System
GSM	Global System for Mobile Communications
ICT	information and communication technology
IDB	Inter-American Development Bank
IR	infrared
IVR	interactive voice response
JMP	Joint Monitoring Programme
LiDAR	light detection and ranging
MDG	Millennium Development Goal
MICS	Multiple Indicator Cluster Surveys
MODIS	Moderate Resolution Imaging Spectroradiometer
MoMo	mobile monitor
MPN	most probable number
NASA	National Aeronautics and Space Administration
NCWSC	Nairobi City Water and Sewerage Company
NDVI	Normalized Differential Vegetation Index
NGO	nongovernmental organization
NRW	non-revenue water
NTU	nephelometric turbidity unit
PA	presence–absence
PLUM	Passive Latrine Use Monitor
QA/QC	quality assurance and quality control
QIS	Qualitative Information System
RSR	really simple reporting

SDG	Sustainable Development Goal
SI	sanitary inspection
SIASAR	*Sistema de Información de Agua y Saneamiento Rural* (Rural Water and Sanitation Information System Initiative)
SIS	sanitary inspection score
SMART	specific, measurable, achievable, relevant, and time-bound
SMS	short message service
TDS	total dissolved solids
TIRS	thermal infrared sensor
TLF	tryptophan-like fluorescence
TTC	thermotolerant coliform
UAV	unmanned aerial vehicle
UN	United Nations
UNICEF	United Nations Children's Fund
USAID	U.S. Agency for International Development
WASH	water, sanitation, and hygiene
WHO	World Health Organization
Wi-Fi	wireless fidelity
WPDx	Water Point Data Exchange
WQR	Water Quality Reporter
WSP	Water and Sanitation Program
WSS	water supply and sanitation

Executive Summary

The Challenge

The United Nations Sustainable Development Goals (SDGs) were announced with fanfare in September 2015. Updating the Millennium Development Goals (MDGs), the 17 SDGs promise to deliver an ambitious range of global impacts, including "End poverty in all its forms everywhere"; "Ensure access to affordable, reliable, sustainable and modern energy for all"; and "Revitalize the global partnership for sustainable development."[1]

The new 2030 Agenda includes water, sanitation, and hygiene (WASH) at its core, with SDG 6 dedicating a commitment to "Ensure availability and sustainable management of water and sanitation for all." Monitoring progress toward this goal will be challenging because direct measures of water and sanitation service quality and use are either expensive or elusive. However, a continued reliance on household surveys poses limitations that likely overstated water access during the MDG period.

The Opportunity

Emergent technologies, methods, and data-sharing platforms are increasingly aligned with impact monitoring. Improved monitoring of water and sanitation interventions may allow more cost-effective and measurable results. In many cases, technologies and methods allow more complete and impartial data in time to allow program improvements.

In this report, we review the landscape of technologies, methods, and approaches that can support and improve on the water and sanitation indicators proposed for SDG targets 6.1, "by 2030, achieve universal and equitable access to safe and affordable drinking water for all," and 6.2, "by 2030, achieve access to adequate and equitable sanitation and hygiene for all and end open defecation, paying special attention to the needs of women and girls and those in vulnerable situations." In some cases, technologies and methods are validated and readily available. In other cases, emergent technologies and approaches hold promise but require further field evaluation and cost reductions.

The World Health Organization and United Nations Children's Fund Joint Monitoring Programme (JMP) for Water and Sanitation has developed proposed indicators for measuring progress toward SDG targets 6.1 and 6.2. In chapter 1, authors with the JMP review the rationale for a continued primary reliance on household surveys and censuses because these data sources are readily available from national statistical offices. However, the JMP has also proposed progressively integrating other data sources, when available, including water quality testing, in situ instrumentation, and Earth observations. Notably, the JMP has proposed a "service ladder" monitoring approach, acknowledging the progressive and nonbinary nature of increased access to safe water and sanitation. The highest rung on the ladder for SDG target 6.1, "universal and equitable access to safe and affordable drinking water for all," focuses on "safely managed drinking water" as measured, when feasible, through direct water quality testing, while lower rungs measure access to "improved" drinking water sources, similar to the approach used in the MDG period. Similarly, hygiene monitoring qualifies "handwashing at home" as the highest service ladder rung, and lower levels examine extra-household services, such as handwashing in schools and health care facilities.

The data and insights gained from these improved monitoring approaches are effective only when leveraged toward improved service delivery in the broader context of maximizing public health. The integration of service ladders and consideration of direct service quality and delivery measures are important steps toward credible and actionable data collection. Building on the JMP's indicator review, in chapter 1 epidemiologists advance the consideration of health impact as a primary driver for water and sanitation monitoring. Reviewing the monitoring approaches used in the MDG period, this chapter highlights the significant gap between "improved" water and sanitation and impacts on health. Constructively, additional measures are proposed including measures of quantity, quality, and sustained access to safe drinking water, including direct and repeated water quality testing, and direct measures of sanitation system integrity and individual use.

Fully reconciling the benefits of measurement quality and integrity provided by direct and repeated or continuous measures of water quality, use, and service delivery with the scalability and cost-effectiveness of household surveys is beyond the scope of this report. However, we advance this discussion through the curation of available and emerging technologies, methods, and systems that may enable cost-effective and reliable water and sanitation monitoring.

In chapter 2, we review water quality monitoring standards applicable to SDG 6 and the JMP's proposed water quality approach, and present methods and technologies for monitoring household and community-level microbial and physiochemical contamination. Typically, the most important water quality measures are in most cases microbial contamination, whereas other contamination may be relevant on a regional or local basis.

Moving beyond the simple classification of a source as improved or unimproved, testing of actual water quality parameters will provide a better measurement of the exposure of users to harmful waterborne constituents. However, testing water at the source provides only a snapshot of water quality at the point of collection and is not representative of the actual water consumed, which may have been contaminated between the source and the point of consumption or at storage. As such, chapter 2 recommends measuring samples that come from a container from which household members actually drink. An array of methods exists for both laboratory and field-based measurement, all of which have their advantages and limitations. However, with any method, proper quality control and quality assurance guidelines should be adhered to when at all possible. When larger or more systematic testing is being undertaken, working with local authorities such as the ministry of health or local environmental protection agency may be appropriate.

Sanitation and hygiene quality measures are, presently, more challenging to measure than water quality. In chapter 3, we review the myriad forms of sanitation and hygiene interventions, and the most relevant measurement characteristics including access, safety, and proper use. An inherent challenge in monitoring sanitation programs is the diversity of behaviors and facilities. Sanitation behaviors encompass defecation, urination, anal cleansing, deposition of children's feces, deposition of cleansing products, separation of solid and liquid waste, fecal sludge management, handwashing, adherence to sanitation facility use, and menstrual hygiene. Different sanitation facilities separate excreta from human contact with varying degrees of efficacy (for example, open defecation versus a flush toilet connected to a sewer system). Finally, there are additional factors that can influence the level of contamination in a sanitation facility, including latrine cleanliness, whether the latrine is shared or private, and the degree to which all members of a household can access the latrine. These layers of behavior, facility type, and facility characteristics interact dynamically and change in time, making it difficult to determine which sanitation features are most important for reducing human exposure to pathogens. Given this complexity, it is important to identify the sanitation outcomes that minimize exposure to pathogens before exploring the best practices and technologies for monitoring those outcomes.

Chapter 3 identifies outcomes that are explicitly or implicitly identified in the SDG target on sanitation and hygiene and the extent to which those outcomes are represented in the proposed service ladders. A variety of innovative practices and technologies are described with specific attention given to their abilities to accurately measure and monitor progress on each outcome.

In chapter 4, we describe some limitations of, and alternatives to, traditional measurement methods for measuring water and sanitation use and behavior. Measurement of adoption and compliance with water and sanitation interventions, such as latrines, water pumps, and water filters, has often relied on surveys and observations. However, surveys and other common methods for assessing behavioral practices are known to have certain methodological shortcomings, including poor correlation between observations and self-reported recall. Survey results can also be affected by errors of interpretation on the part of the informant or the enumerator. Data missing because of participant absences or failure to follow up is another source of systematic bias. Additionally, it is known that the act of surveying or observation can itself impact later behavior, a phenomenon known as reactivity or the Hawthorne effect. Structured observation, an alternative to relying on reported behavior in response to surveys, has also been shown to cause reactivity in the target population. Finally, the subjectivity of the outcome studied can strongly influence reporting bias. In chapter 4, we highlight these challenges while proposing direct and indirect measures of behavior and use that can better estimate progress toward SDG 6.

Emergent technologies, including water meters, water pump sensors, and latrine motion detectors can improve the objectivity and continuity of data collection. Satellite-based remote sensing and sensors linked to the Internet of Things can be aligned with smartphone-based surveys and online "big data" tools. These technologies and services are reviewed in chapters 5 and 6, and may offer improvements in the collection of, and action on, data from water and sanitation programs.

The term "remote sensing" usually describes the collection of data by satellites. In most cases, "remote" refers to spectral imagery collected by cameras and other spectral instruments across a broad range of wavelengths. In the case of Earth observation, satellites take spectral data reflected from the atmosphere and the Earth's surface. Interpretation of these data (often represented as imagery) requires an understanding of spectral data and physical properties of the Earth and its atmosphere. Interpretation often also requires calibration against data collected on the Earth's surface or in the atmosphere directly—data from sensors that are in situ rather than remote.

In situ instrumentation technologies vary from flow meters and water quality sensors to motion detectors installed in latrines. These sensor technologies can be used either operationally or within a statistical sampling frame. Data can be logged locally for manual retrieval or transmitted over short range to nearby enumerators, or to remote operators and researchers over Wi-Fi, cellular, and satellite networks. Some instrumentation is in common use, while other technologies are emerging. However, given the remote and power-constrained environments and the high degree of variability between fixed infrastructure—including age, materials, quality, servicing, and functionality—any electronic sensor–based solution often either is custom engineered or compensates for these complexities through analytics. For example, a conventional flow meter designed for a rural borehole water distribution scheme would have to address pipe diameter, material, pressure, depth, thread type, and other characteristics that require custom engineering and plumbing, whereas a nonintrusive ultrasonic flow meter may be more easily adapted for a variety of water schemes.

Cellular phone–based data collection with online analytics and dissemination is a rapidly growing field for water and sanitation programs. The field of mobile surveys provides a user-friendly platform to easily collect data using a mobile platform rather than a paper-based survey. The mobile platform additionally allows for Global Positioning System (GPS) coordinates, barcode scanning, and photos to be easily associated with a particular sample. The ability to look at photos and confirm GPS coordinates creates both ease of data analysis and surveyor accountability. In chapter 6, a number of electronic data collection and dissemination tools used in WASH programs are reviewed.

Looking Forward

Each of these myriad monitoring and evaluation methods has its own advantages and limitations. It is often beneficial to leverage more than one method to get a fuller picture of water and sanitation service delivery and adoption behavior. Combined methodologies reinforce the advantages, while also addressing the limitations, of the individual monitoring techniques that compose them. Surveys, ethnographies, and direct observation give context to electronic sensor readings that may be more continuous and objective. Overall, combined methodologies can provide a more comprehensive and instructive depiction of WASH usage.

Some of the technologies and methods presented in this report are well established, whereas others hold promise but require extensive field-testing and validation, commercialization, and scaling. Because applications vary widely, we have not attempted to directly compare costs between methods and technologies. Likewise, it is beyond the scope of our report to compare the relative value or reliability of different methods. Instead, we present a menu of options for policy makers, program implementers, and auditors to consider when designing impact measurement efforts.

Note

1. For the complete list of Sustainable Development Goals, see the United Nations SDG website, http://www.un.org/sustainabledevelopment/sustainable-development-goals/.

CHAPTER 1

A Review of WASH Monitoring Indicators

Introduction

During the Millennium Development Goal (MDG) period, international monitoring of water, sanitation, and hygiene (WASH) services in developing countries relied predominantly on household surveys identifying access to "improved" and "unimproved" services. However, these indicators fell short of the key health-based conditions that the MDG water and sanitation targets sought to encourage. Overly simplistic metrics used to monitor progress on important health and development goals can be misleading—monitoring that relies on poor indicators can exaggerate progress. Additionally, inadequate assessments of environmental health interventions can undermine the proper allocation of scarce resources for advancing intended goals. The beginning of the Sustainable Development Goal (SDG) period offers an opportunity to learn from these limitations to better align indicators and measures with intended outcomes. In this chapter, the current indicators proposed by the World Health Organization/United Nations Children's Fund (WHO/UNICEF) Joint Monitoring Programme (JMP) for Water and Sanitation are reviewed, followed by a summary of limitations during the MDG period, which can inform improved SDG monitoring. These new indicators address in part the MDG limitations while balancing the likely availability of robust data sources. In subsequent chapters, technologies and methods are reviewed that meet and may exceed these indicator data requirements.

Proposed WASH Indicators for the SDGs
by Tom Slaymaker

The WHO/UNICEF JMP has been identified as the data custodian for the SDG 6.1 and 6.2 targets. Since 2011, the JMP has facilitated international consultations to develop proposals for monitoring the progressive elimination of inequalities in access to different levels of drinking water, sanitation, and hygiene services.

In this section, we review the current indicators and rationale proposed by the JMP for SDG targets 6.1 and 6.2.

Background and Guiding Principles

In a report to the United Nations (UN) General Assembly, the Open Working Group on SDGs proposed a framework of 17 SDGs covering a range of drivers across the three pillars of sustainable development.[1] The Open Working Group proposal includes a dedicated goal on water and sanitation comprising six technical targets (below). This chapter covers indicators for monitoring target 6.1 on drinking water and 6.2 on sanitation and hygiene.

Targets 6.1 and 6.2 seek to address the unfinished business and shortcomings of MDG target 7c and call for universal access to drinking water, sanitation, and hygiene. Targets 6. 2 and 6.3 expand the framework beyond the use of sanitation facilities to cover the full sanitation chain and underscore the importance of treating wastewater, which is a dominant cause of water pollution and deteriorating water quality (see box 1.1 for more information on SDG 6).

Box 1.1 SDG 6: Ensure Availability and Sustainable Management of Water and Sanitation for All

6.1. By 2030, achieve universal and equitable access to safe and affordable **drinking water** for all

6.2. By 2030, achieve access to adequate and equitable **sanitation and hygiene** for all **and end open defecation**, paying special attention to the needs of women and girls and those in vulnerable situations

6.3. By 2030, improve **water quality** by reducing pollution, eliminating dumping and minimizing release of hazardous chemicals and materials, halving the proportion of untreated **wastewater** and substantially increasing recycling and safe reuse globally

6.4. By 2030, substantially increase **water-use efficiency** across all sectors and ensure **sustainable withdrawals** and supply of freshwater to address water scarcity and substantially reduce the number of people suffering from water scarcity

6.5. By 2030, implement **integrated water resources management** at all levels, including through transboundary cooperation as appropriate

6.6. By 2020, protect and restore **water-related ecosystems**, including mountains, forests, wetlands, rivers, aquifers and lakes

6a. By 2030, expand international cooperation and capacity-building support to developing countries in water- and sanitation-related activities and programmes, including water harvesting, desalination, water efficiency, wastewater treatment, recycling and reuse technologies

6b. Support and strengthen the participation of local communities in improving water and sanitation management

Source: Sustainable Development Knowledge Platform, https://sustainabledevelopment.un.org/sdg6.
Note: Emphasis added.

Criteria for Indicator Selection and Data Sources

The foremost purpose of global monitoring is to provide evidence for policy making; monitoring must therefore be action-oriented, measuring progress objectively for the global community and providing guidance on global investments. Indicators proposed in this document have been selected on the basis of the following criteria so that they

- Are prominent in the monitoring of major international declarations to which (all) UN member states have agreed, or are identified through international mechanisms such as reference or interagency groups as a priority indicator in specific program areas;
- Are scientifically robust, useful, accessible, understandable, and SMART (specific, measurable, achievable, relevant, and time-bound);
- Are relevant as assessed by UN member states;
- Exhibit a strong track record, preferably supported by experience and an international database;
- Are used by countries in the monitoring of national plans and programs and are tried and tested by individual countries, by individual regions, or globally as part of intergovernmental processes;
- Are methodologically sound and easy to understand and communicate;
- Offer the possibility for aggregation/disaggregation; and
- Are universal but adaptable to local conditions.

Global monitoring requires timely and reliable data gathered in a cost-effective manner. For example, the JMP relies primarily on household surveys and censuses conducted by national statistical offices. These serve multiple sectors, are known for their quality and reliability, and provide data at minimal additional cost. Household surveys and censuses will therefore remain the primary source of data for monitoring targets 6.1 and 6.2 as well as the domestic wastewater part of 6.3 in the SDG period (see table 1.1). But, in order to address the ambition of the SDG targets, other data sources will be progressively integrated and will include administrative sources and regulators as well as other novel but highly cost-effective sources such as in situ sensors, water quality testing, and earth observations.

The next section outlines the latest proposed methods and indicators for estimating progress in relation to proposed SDG targets on drinking water, sanitation, hygiene, and wastewater. Whereas some of the indicators identified are already well established and can be monitored immediately, others are relatively new and will need to be developed over the short, medium, or long term. Global and regional estimates can be made on the basis of the limited data already available, but indicator availability at the country level is expected to increase throughout the SDG period.

Proposed Indicators and Monitoring Framework

This section identifies the key indicators that could be used for monitoring the proposed SDG targets in all countries. For each target, water and sanitation

Table 1.1 SDG Target 6.1 and Target 6.2 Definition, Data Sources, and Disaggregation

SDG target	Indicator	Definition	Data sources and measurability	Disaggregation	Timeline
6.1. Safely managed water	Percentage of population using safely managed drinking water services	Population using an improved drinking water source that is located on premises, available when needed, and free of fecal (and priority chemical) contamination. Improved water sources: piped water into dwelling, yard, or plot; public taps or standpipes; boreholes or tubewells; protected dug wells, protected springs, and rainwater.	Household surveys can provide data on improved water on premises as well as availability when needed and freedom from contamination via direct water quality testing. Administrative sources including drinking water regulators can provide data on compliance with standards for water quality and availability.	Urban/rural Wealth Affordability Others	Elements from household surveys can be reported immediately. Safety/regulation will initially be estimated globally and regionally, and progressively at country level.
6.2. Safely managed sanitation	Percentage of population using safely managed sanitation services	Population using an improved sanitation facility that is not shared with other households and where excreta are safely disposed in situ or treated off-site. This is a dual-purpose indicator covering the domestic part of wastewater treatment of 6.3.	Household surveys can provide info on types of sanitation facilities and disposal in situ. Administrative, population, and environmental data can be used to estimate safe disposal/treatment of excreta.	Urban/rural Wealth Affordability Others	Elements from household surveys can be reported in the short term. Excreta management will initially be estimated globally and regionally, and progressively at country level.
6.2. Hand washing at home	Percentage of population with handwashing facilities with soap and water at home	Population with a handwashing facility with soap and water in the household.	Household surveys	Urban/rural Wealth Affordability Others	Immediate

Source: WHO/UNICEF 2017.

Note: Top row is proposed Sustainable Development Goal indicator; following rows are part of global reporting "ladder" used by the Joint Monitoring Programme.

"ladders" are also proposed to illustrate progressive improvement in both service levels and monitoring over time and across countries at different stages of development. These ladders and an extensive review of the indicators are available from the JMP website[2] (WHO/UNICEF 2015a).

Detailed Methodology: Safely Managed Drinking Water Services

The proposed indicator of "safely managed drinking water services" comprises four elements:

1. Improved drinking water source that is
2. Located on premises,
3. Available when needed, and
4. Compliant with fecal (and priority chemical) standards

The first three of these can be measured through integrated household surveys, and data collection will be similar to that for the "improved drinking water" indicator used for MDG monitoring. Data for these elements are immediately available for over 100 countries, although questions on availability are not usually explicitly asked in household surveys but implied when households identify their main source of drinking water. Household surveys can also provide information on water quality testing as direct measurement of water quality is increasingly adopted as a module in surveys. Regulatory authorities also collect information on the proportion of populations accessing different types of regulated water services, and the extent to which such services provide water that is available when needed, is located on premises, and meets quality standards.

Proposed Indicators and Monitoring Framework for Sanitation and Hygiene

The JMP defines "safely managed sanitation services" as population using an improved sanitation facility that is not shared with other households and where excreta are safely disposed of in situ or treated off-site (for MDG monitoring purposes, "improved" sanitation facility means flush or pour flush toilets to sewer systems, septic tanks or pit latrines, ventilated improved pit latrines, pit latrines with a slab, and composting toilets—the same categories as improved sources of drinking water).

Household surveys and censuses provide data on use of types of improved sanitation facilities listed above. The percentage of the population using safely managed sanitation services can be calculated by combining data on the proportion of the population using different types of improved sanitation facilities with estimates of the proportion of fecal waste that is safely disposed of in situ or transported to a designated place for safe disposal or treatment. Similar "safety factors" representing the proportion of waste that is safely disposed of in situ or transported to a designated place are required to estimate the proportion of wastewater that is safely treated under target 6.3.

One of the main critiques of the water and sanitation targets in the MDGs is that hygiene was not considered despite its clear links with health and with other economic and social benefits. Hygiene behaviors are very distinct from sanitation and management of fecal wastes, and require separate indicators. Accordingly, the JMP proposes handwashing at home with soap as a core indicator for tracking target 6.2. The JMP also proposes two supporting indicators: (i) handwashing in schools and health facilities, and (ii) menstrual hygiene management in schools and health facilities. Data on hygiene in schools and health care facilities will be collected through a combination of institutional surveys and sector management information systems. JMP recognizes also that food hygiene is important, and will engage with evolving methods to measure food hygiene in the household.

Household Surveys within SDG Monitoring Indicators

The WASH MDG framework relied primarily on measurements collected through household surveys. As such, the institutional knowledge, efforts, and successes built and achieved under the MDG time frame remain relevant, and contribute building blocks of SDG monitoring. Appendix A of this report discusses how the MDG framework will be built into the SDG monitoring. In appendix A, we first review the long-collected measurements used in MDG monitoring. Their continued collection remains fundamental for future monitoring under the SDGs. Second, we specify how other measurements collected during the MDG time frame, but not critical to MDG monitoring, now make their way formally into SDG monitoring. These first two groups of measurements can be understood to meet all eight criteria for indicator selection and data sources listed in this chapter. Third, we outline the category of household survey–based measurements that are critical to SDG monitoring but that are only recently being rolled out for widespread collection. All these elements of SDG monitoring that come from household surveys are noted in table 1.1 as "can be reported immediately" or "can be reported in the short term" because the technology is fully ready and either widespread historically or being rolled out. Last, appendix A closes with a review of some main challenges and opportunities in the full rollout of these household survey components of SDG measurements.

Improving Safe Water and Sanitation Monitoring for Health Gains
by Thomas Clasen

In early 2012, WHO and UNICEF made an important announcement: "The world has met the Millennium Development Goal (MDG) target of halving the proportion of people without sustainable access to safe drinking water, well in advance of the MDG 2015 deadline" (WHO and UNICEF 2012). Major news organizations heralded the accomplishment. The editors of *The Lancet* (2012) used the occasion to draw attention to underachievement of other MDG targets but still acknowledged the water announcement as "some good news to celebrate." There was little celebrating, however, among many who work at the intersection of water and health. This is because the way progress was measured on the MDG water target—by counting those who have access to "improved water supplies"—did not fully address water quality, quantity, and sustainable access—key components of the target that are fundamental to human health.

Similarly, even the stated shortfall in the sanitation goal—2.1 billion people gained access to improved sanitation since 1990, while another 2.5 billion still lack access to improved sanitation—exaggerates actual progress. This is due to a misalignment between the MDG sanitation goal and the manner in which progress toward that goal was measured under international monitoring.

As monitoring programs are being developed for the new water and sanitation targets under the SDG, it is important that they actually address the key aspects of WASH interventions that optimize the potential contribution to human health, in particular reduced waterborne disease.

SDG Water Monitoring Review

Over the years, considerable efforts have been undertaken to expand the scope of international water quality monitoring in order to address the key components of quality, quantity, and sustainable access that are vital to improve health. The third edition of WHO's *Guidelines for Drinking Water Quality* recommends a more comprehensive approach that addresses quality, coverage, quantity, continuity, and cost (WHO 1997). A health-based approach using water service levels was proposed in 2003, and a human rights–based approach was adopted in 2008 (Kayser et al. 2013).

There is increasing recognition of the need for a more comprehensive "service quality" or "service ladder" approach, as proposed by the JMP, that accounts for the different levels of service provided by various drinking water and sanitation facilities, and their associated benefits (Bartram et al. 2014). Bartram and colleagues argue that, at a minimum, this system should distinguish piped, household connections from other types of improved water supplies. They also recommend that water source functionality and reliability should be part of the analysis. Finally, for households without access to reliable household-level piped supplies, they recommend some measure of the safety of household drinking water storage methods, but it is not clear if this would constitute some type of water safety plan compliance or actual testing of water quality. Also unclear is whether this ladder would somehow incorporate measures of water quantity or actual use.

Perhaps more important to comprehensive water quality monitoring, however, are the indicators for the SDG 6 targets. A recent review has described the use of a large variety of indicators to assess water source/technology type (including whether categorized as "improved," "unimproved," community source, or on-plot water); accessibility; water safety (quality and sanitary risk); water quantity, reliability, or continuity; affordability; and equity (Kayser et al. 2013). Although the review explored the potential for combining these indicators into a comprehensive framework, it concluded that the scientific basis for doing so was still lacking and that further research was necessary.

Innovations in WASH Impact Measures • http://dx.doi.org/10.1596/978-1-4648-1197-5

SDG Sanitation Monitoring Review

WHO and UNICEF have published indicators for the SDG sanitation target that address many of the shortcomings of the MDG target. A significant improvement over the MDGs is the inclusion of the complete sanitation system chain. The new targets include the three main aspects of the MDGs—system integrity, coverage, and use—and also incorporate all services and infrastructures from the point of excretion to end treatment/disposal under the monitoring agenda, which will be a major challenge in determining indicators for assessment. By including "for all," the target mandates that, for sanitation systems and services to be included under the definition of "improved" sanitation, they must be available at all times to all people, no matter age, gender, disability status, or income level. Incorporation of child feces disposal into the definition of open defecation requires that all feces, from both child and adult no matter the age, be disposed of in a safe and hygienic manner, whether in an improved sanitation facility or in a treatment system. Last, the addition of special attention to women, girls, and those in "vulnerable populations" requires that additional measures be met to provide for the sanitation needs of women and girls with regard to water collection and special sanitation requirements, as well as to ensure that all people in "refugee camps, detention centers, mass gatherings, and pilgrimages" have adequate sanitation.

Although the SDG sanitation target and its expanded interpretation address the major factors that are necessary to advance health, the SDG indicators fall short in creating a means of directly and comprehensively assessing progress toward the target (WHO/UNICEF 2015b).

Under the current proposal, "basic sanitation" will be measured using a binary definition of improved/unimproved sanitation facility (WHO/UNICEF 2015b). WHO and UNICEF define open defecation as the "percentage of population that practices open defecation." In relation to "sustainable," the indicator is proposed as the "percentage of population using a safely-managed sanitation facility that reliably provides expected levels of service, and is subject to robust regulation and a verified risk management plan." Inequality will also be assessed by disaggregating the data on the basis of various factors, including urban/rural location, wealth quintiles, subnational regions, informal settlements, sex, age, or disability status (WHO/UNICEF 2015b). Last, the JMP will partner with Global Expanded Monitoring Initiative, a global monitoring program, to measure indicators for target 6.2. "Safely managed" sanitation will be measured as the "percentage of population using a basic sanitation facility where excreta are safely disposed in-situ or safely transported and treated off-site" (WHO/UNICEF 2015b).

Sanitation coverage and use will be measured only at the household level, providing no conclusion on community, neighborhood, or city-level access and use. The negative impacts of incomplete sanitation coverage at the community level have been seen in field studies and systematic reviews (Moraes, Cancio, and Cairncross 2004; Barreto et al. 2007; Geruso and Spears 2015). A study of city-wide sanitation improvements in Salvador, Brazil, saw overall reductions in the prevalence of diarrhea by 21 percent; in high-risk areas with high baseline prevalence, the reduction was 43 percent (Barreto et al. 2007). Use will once again be assessed in response to household surveys that ask respondents which type of facility they "usually use," presenting the same problems discussed above with respect to the MDGs.

One clear advance of the proposed indicators is the focus on fecal sludge management. The indicator defines "safely managed sanitation" as systems whose fecal waste is transported through a sewer to a designated location, is collected from systems by a process that limits human contact and is transported to a designated location, or undergoes at minimum secondary treatment or "primary treatment with long ocean outfall for sewerage" or is treated at a "managed disposal site" or wastewater treatment plant or "stored on site until…safe to handle and re-use" (WHO/UNICEF 2015b). This indicator is designed to encompass essential services and operational requirements for public health benefits (Feachem et al. 1983; Shuval 2003; Escamilla et al. 2013). At the same time, the indicator does not evaluate the integrity of the system or services, nor is there consideration of sustainability.

Notes

1. For the complete list of Sustainable Development Goals, see the United Nations SDG website, http://www.un.org/sustainabledevelopment/sustainable-development-goals/.

2. For more information, see https://washdata.org.

References

Barreto, M. L., B. Genser, A. Strina, M. G. Teixeira, A. M. Assis, R. F. Rego, C. A. Teles, M. S. Prado, S. M. Matos, D. N. Santos, L. A. dos Santos, and S. Cairncross. 2007. "Effect of City-Wide Sanitation Programme on Reduction in Rate of Childhood Diarrhoea in Northeast Brazil: Assessment by Two Cohort Studies." *The Lancet* 370 (9599): 1622–28.

Bartram, J., C. Brockelhurst, M. B. Fisher, R. Luyendijk, T. Wardlaw, and B. Gordon. 2014. "Global Monitoring of Water Supply and Sanitation: History, Methods, and Future Challenges." *International Journal of Environmental Research and Public Health* 11 (8): 8137–65.

Escamilla, V., P. S. K. Knappett, M. Yunus, P. K. Streatfield, and M. Emch. 2013. "Influence of Latrine Proximity and Type on Tubewell Water Quality and Diarrheal Disease in Bangladesh." *Annals of the Association of American Geographers* 103 (2): 299–308.

Feachem, R. G., D. J. Bradley, H. Garelick, and D. D. Mara. 1983. *Sanitation and Disease: Health Aspects of Wastewater and Excreta Management.* World Bank Studies in Water Supply and Sanitation. Washington, DC: World Bank.

Geruso, M., and D. Spears. 2015. "Neighborhood Sanitation and Infant Mortality." NBER Working Paper 21184, National Bureau of Economic Research, Cambridge, MA.

Kayser, G. L., P. Moriarty, C. Fonseca, and J. Bartram. 2013. "Domestic Water Service Delivery Indicators and Frameworks for Monitoring, Evaluation, Policy and Planning:

A Review." *International Journal of Environmental Research and Public Health* 10 (10): 4812–35.

Moraes, L. R., J. A. Cancio, and S. Cairncross. 2004. "Impact of Drainage and Sewerage on Intestinal Nematode Infections in Poor Urban Areas in Salvador, Brazil." *Transactions of the Royal Society of Tropical Medicine and Hygiene* 98 (4): 197–204.

Shuval, H. 2003. "Estimating the Global Burden of Thalassogenic Diseases: Human Infectious Diseases Caused by Wastewater Pollution of the Marine Environment." *Journal of Water and Health* 1 (2): 53–64.

The Lancet. 2012. "Progress in Sanitation Needed for Neglected Tropical Diseases." *The Lancet* 379 (9820): 978.

WHO (World Health Organization). 1997. *Guidelines for Drinking-Water Quality: Surveillance and Control of Community Supplies.* Geneva: World Health Organization.

WHO (World Health Organization) and UNICEF (United Nations Children's Fund). 2012. "Millennium Development Goal Drinking Water Target." News Release, March 6. http://www.who.int/mediacentre/news/releases/2012/drinking_water _20120306/en/.

WHO/UNICEF (WHO/UNICEF Joint Monitoring Programme for Water and Sanitation). 2015a. *Methodological Note: Proposed Indicator Framework for Monitoring SDG Targets on Drinking-Water, Sanitation, Hygiene and Wastewater.* Geneva: WHO and UNICEF.

———. 2015b. *JMP Green Paper: Global Monitoring of Water, Sanitation and Hygiene Post-2015.* Geneva: WHO and UNICEF.

———. 2017. *Progress on Drinking Water, Sanitation, and Hygiene: 2017 Update and SDG Baselines.* Geneva: WHO and UNICEF.

Water Quality Monitoring

Christina Barstow

Introduction

In this chapter, we review the technologies and methods available for measuring water quality—an important indicator of safe water service delivery. As described in chapter 2, the Joint Monitoring Programme indicator for Sustainable Development Goal 6 describes safely managed water as the "population using an improved drinking water source, which is located on premises, available when needed and free of fecal (and priority chemical) contamination." On a global level, priority chemical contaminants of interest are typically fluoride and arsenic.

Although classification of water sources as "improved" versus "unimproved" can streamline a monitoring effort, an "improved" source may still be contaminated, either from source contamination itself or during the process of collection and storage of water before the water has been consumed. In contrast to the relatively simple and low-cost survey-based process of "improved" versus "unimproved" water source classification, measurement of contaminants can be more expensive and time consuming and require specialized equipment and training.

Water Quality Guidelines and Specifications

The World Health Organization (WHO) has developed relevant water quality guidelines and monitoring documents. Specifically, the *Guidelines for Drinking-Water Quality* provide recommendations to manage risk of waterborne contaminants (WHO 2011b). The *Guidelines* describe recommendations where possible according to health-based targets calculated from a tolerable burden of disease, using the metric disability adjusted life years. From an acute perspective, pathogens are the primary concern; and fecally derived pathogens set the basis for the targets. The *Guidelines* recommend that drinking water contain no fecal indicator organisms but additionally classify risk on the basis of a log scale of coliforms per 100 milliliters (table 2.1). *Escherichia coli* (*E. coli*) or thermotolerant coliforms (TTCs) are recommended as fecal indicator organisms and commonly used

Table 2.1 Microbial Risk Classifications

Concentration (CFU/100 mL)	Risk classification
<1	Low
1–10	Intermediate
11–100	High
>100	Very high

Note: CFU = colony forming unit.

because of their high numbers in polluted waters, relative ease of administering the test method, and the general familiarity with this method within the water quality sector.

From a chronic perspective, chemical constituents are the primary concern. Chemical contaminants can be introduced from a variety of sources including those that are naturally occurring and industrial activities, agricultural activities, and other anthropogenic sources. Guideline values are set for a wide range of chemical contaminants whereby the value is the limit where significant health risk is not realized over a lifetime. Although the *Guidelines* outline hundreds of chemical constituents, only those that are known to be a risk in a particular region are usually measured regularly. A common example is arsenic contamination in some regions of Bangladesh and India (WHO 2011b).

WHO provides additional guidance in *Evaluating Household Water Treatment Options: Health-Based Targets for Microbiological Performance Specifications* (hereafter, the *Specifications*) (WHO 2011a). Although it relates to household water treatment, the document also outlines important guidance for technology-specific water treatment options. Community water treatment versus household water treatment is discussed further in the next section to provide more context for the use of the *Specifications*. Additionally, the *Specifications* provide guidance only for microbial contamination because most household water treatment options target only microbial pathogens according to acute health-based targets. The *Specifications* outline reduction values for reference pathogens for bacteria, viruses, and protozoa. Reference pathogens include *Campylobacter* for bacteria, rotavirus for viruses, and *Cryptosporidium* for protozoa. A log reduction value for each reference pathogen can be measured for a particular household water treatment technology, which is then categorized as highly protective, protective, or interim, as shown in table 2.2 (WHO 2011a).

Given the large number of possible chemical contaminants and the impracticality of measuring all constituents, WHO developed a guidance document to help identify priority chemicals within a specific country or program context entitled *Chemical Safety of Drinking Water: Assessing Priorities for Risk Management* (WHO 2012). *Chemical Safety* outlines a strategy whereby priority chemicals are identified through assessment of existing data sources in five source categories: (i) naturally occurring chemicals, (ii) chemicals from agricultural activities, (iii) chemicals from human settlements, (iv) chemicals from industrial activities, and (v) chemicals from water treatment and distribution. *Chemical Safety* pays

Table 2.2 WHO Microbial Reduction Standard for Household Water Treatment

	Log_{10} reduction required		
Target	Bacteria	Viruses	Protozoa
Highly protective	>4	>5	>4
Protective	>2	>3	>2
Interim	Achieves "protective" for two classes of pathogens and results in health gains		

Source: WHO 2011a.
Note: WHO = World Health Organization.

particular focus to a small list of constituents that have been found worldwide, identifying and describing fluoride, arsenic, selenium, nitrate, iron, manganese, and lead. Fluoride, arsenic, and selenium are naturally occurring compounds usually found in groundwater. Nitrate, which can also be naturally occurring, is a key constituent of fertilizers and is often associated with agricultural activities. Iron and manganese, although not considered to be harmful, can cause water discoloration, which often leads to discontinued water use among consumers. Last, lead is identified because of its presence in many distribution networks in plumbing materials. In this chapter, the frequently identified chemicals of fluoride, arsenic, selenium, nitrate, iron, and manganese will be discussed more in the water quality measurement section. We do not discuss lead because of the low likelihood of its occurrence in the developing countries context (WHO 2012). WHO guidelines for the chemicals identified here are summarized in table 2.3.

Another frequently monitored chemical is the free chlorine residual. Chlorine does not occur naturally but rather is often added as a disinfectant during the water treatment process. Management of chlorine residual requires a balance between maintaining an adequate level of chlorine within the system and avoiding the creation of disinfection byproducts when chlorine reacts with natural organic matter. When chlorine is used as the primary disinfection mechanism, the minimum recommended concentration is 0.2 mg/L of free chlorine residual throughout the distribution and in water samples from household water storage vessels. Disinfection byproducts are not often considered in a developing community context because chlorine levels are usually low, but a maximum of 5 mg/L of free chlorine is recommended.

Consideration is also warranted for several operational parameters, mainly pH, total dissolved solids (TDS), and turbidity. Although these parameters don't directly affect health, they can be important during water treatment processes and in the distribution system. pH is often measured through several stages including disinfection with chlorine. It is recommended that pH be between 6.5 and 8.5. High values of TDS can cause scaling in water pipes and an unpleasant taste to consumers. WHO recommends TDS levels of less than 600 mg/L whereas the U.S. Environmental Protection Agency (EPA) recommends 500 mg/L (EPA 2016b). Levels exceeding 1,000 mg/L become significantly unpleasant to consumers. Finally, turbidity is important because consumers do not want visibly cloudy or "dirty" water and because particles can hinder the disinfection process.

Table 2.3 WHO Microbial and Chemical Contamination Guidelines

Parameter	Permissible level according to WHO
Total chlorine	5 mg/L
Free chlorine	0.5 mg/L
E. coli	Not present
Temperature	15 °C
pH	6.5–8.5
Salinity	1,500 mg/L
TDS	n.a.
Conductivity	1,000 us/cm
Total hardness	500 mg/l
Color	15 Platinum-Cobalt scale units
Turbidity	5 NTU (84.12 cm)
Nitrates	50 mg/L
Nitrites	3 mg/L
Arsenic	0.01 mg/L
Fluoride	1.5 mg/L
Sulfate	400 mg/L
Manganese	0.4 mg/L
Iron	0.3 mg/L

Source: WHO 2011b.

Note: n.a. = not applicable; NTU = nephelometric turbidity unit; TDS = total dissolved solids; WHO = World Health Organization.

For example, with ultraviolet disinfection, microbes can be hidden from irradiation, impairing the disinfection mechanism. It is generally recommended that turbidity levels be maintained at less than one nephelometric turbidity unit (NTU), while lower levels are preferable. Other operational parameters such as temperature, hardness, and dissolved oxygen concentration, to name a few, should also be measured according to context-specific source water and drinking water treatment needs (WHO 2011b).

While this chapter provides important minimum guidance for water quality measurement, it is essential to recognize the importance of national- and local-level standards and practices. The *Guidelines* document intentionally does not promote an international standard and supports the development of a local risk management strategy. Although the parameters outlined here should be considered, drinking water safety should be assessed and monitored according to context-specific needs and constraints, taking into consideration local capacity and resources.

Water Quality Measurement Methods

Moving beyond the simple classification of a source as improved or unimproved, testing of actual water quality parameters will provide a better measurement of the exposure of harmful waterborne constituents to users. Further, testing water only at the source provides a snapshot of water quality at the point of collection but does not represent the quality of the water actually consumed.

Water may be contaminated between the source and the point of consumption or at storage. As such, it is recommended that water quality be measured using a sample from a typical drinking water container. An array of methods exists for both laboratory and field-based measurement, all of which have their advantages and limitations. As with any method, proper quality assurance and quality control (QA/QC) guidelines should be adhered to when possible. Many of the methods cited in this section include QA/QC measures such as insuring controls and blanks are included in the testing procedure and analysis. When larger or more systematic testing is being undertaken, using local authorities such as the ministry of health or local environmental protection agency may be appropriate.

Laboratory Methods

Several guidelines and methods documents exist that outline standardized and accepted protocols for measurement of water parameters. The most common resource is the *Standard Methods for the Examination of Water and Wastewater* (Rice et al. 2012), currently in its 22nd edition. Additionally, the EPA publishes the "Clean Water Act Analytical Methods" (EPA 2016a), and the International Standards Organization has developed a standards catalogue (ISO 2016).

Microbial Methods

Bacteria. E. coli is the most common indicator used in laboratory settings to determine bacterial contamination. Many methods are outlined in the guidelines documents to quantify *E. coli* contamination. Three of the more common methods are described below (Rice et al. 2012).

1. **Presence–absence (PA)**: The PA is a simple test wherein a water sample is combined with a pre-made growth medium and incubated. Growth of *E. coli* can be detected visually using either color changes or detection of fluorescence when the sample is placed under an ultraviolet light. The PA test is useful for monitoring quality according to the WHO guideline and where quantification of *E. coli* levels is not required.

2. **Most probable number (MPN)**: The MPN method is similar to the PA method but with the ability to obtain an estimate of the *E. coli* concentration in the sample. The MPN method involves splitting the sample into multiple test volumes, each of which detects the presence or absence of *E. coli*. High levels of *E. coli* can be detected through dilution or the use of many small volumes. The most probable concentration of *E. coli* can be calculated on the basis of the test volumes in which *E. coli* are detected.

3. **Colony counting**: The primary technique used to obtain actual *E. coli* concentration is the membrane filtration method. A water sample is filtered, by vacuum, through a membrane filter, which is then placed on a nutrient medium and incubated. The concentration of *E. coli* can then be directly

counted as the number of colonies present. Membrane filtration usually involves a more complex procedure than the MPN method but allows the user to get a more precise count of *E. coli* contamination. In addition to membrane filtration, it is possible to detect high levels of *E. coli* using dip slides or plates that typically allow for the enumeration of *E. coli* in a 1–2 mL sample of water.

Viruses. Coliphages are often used as the reference pathogen of viral contamination from fecal sources (Harwood, Jiang, and Sobsey 2015). Coliphages are viruses that infect and replicate inside a bacteria host. Testing can be conducted with a variety of coliphages, but commonly the MS2 and phiX174 coliphages are used with *E. coli* as their host bacteria.

Several methods exist for the enumeration of coliphages. A frequently used method, the single agar layer method, takes the sample and mixes it with the host bacteria specific to the coliphage and media for the host to grow on. Samples are spread onto plates and then incubated whereby the concentration of the coliphage can be read as the number of plaques on the plate. The *E. coli* bacteria exist in the sample at a high concentration to create a layer of *E. coli* whereby plaque formation are zones where there is *E. coli* absence (EPA 2001).

Protozoa. As mentioned previously, *Cryptosporidium* is used as the reference pathogen for protozoa testing. A common laboratory methodology is EPA Method 1623. In this method, water samples are filtered, and the materials left on the filter are eluted. The elute is centrifuged to pelletize the oocysts and cysts and remove the extraneous materials. The oocysts and cysts are then made paramagnetic to further remove extraneous materials. Fluorescence and differential interference contrast microscopy are then used for quantitative analysis of the *Cryptosporidium* (EPA 2005).

Chemical and Operational Parameters Methods

Measurement of chemical parameters is easily performed through the use of standard laboratory instruments. The six priority chemicals (fluoride, arsenic, selenium, nitrate, iron, and manganese) highlighted in this report as well as chlorine can all be measured through a variety of photometers, colorimeters, and spectrophotometers. A reagent is added to the sample and inserted into the instruments. The chemical concentration is then determined by the intensity of light, absorbance of specific color bands, or transmittance as a function of wavelengths, depending on which type of meter is used. Each instrument will provide its advantages in relation to detection limits and ease of use. Operational parameters are similarly easily measured using instrumentation. pH is measured using a pH meter where an electrode is inserted into the water and the pH is determined by the meter. TDS meters report the concentration by means of measuring the electrical conductivity of the water sample. Finally, turbidity is measured using a turbidimeter, which determines the obstruction of light transmittance through a sample. Meters are available from Hach, Palintest, Lovibond, Extech, Hanna Instruments, Industrial Test Systems, and DelAgua, to name only a few of the possible vendors. Further methods are additionally outlined in the *Standard Methods for the Examination of Water and Wastewater* (Rice et al. 2012).

Field-Based Methods

Although laboratory measurement provides a controlled environment with standardized equipment, it is often challenging or cost prohibitive to analyze samples in the laboratory. For most microbial measurements, only a short period of time can pass before the sample needs to be analyzed because of the inherent nature of microbes growing and dying within water. Bringing a sample back to a laboratory from a remote location will often not meet this time restraint (preferably less than six hours) and risks additional contamination while the sample is being transported. Additionally, standard procedures would require transport of samples on ice, which can greatly complicate logistics. Furthermore, in the case of testing water treatment technologies, it is especially important to recognize that the laboratory testing environment may not represent actual field conditions. A variety of scenarios in which the water testing technology is being misused or poorly maintained, or in which the surroundings provide additional contamination pathways, could provide different results than laboratory-based methods.

Microbial Methods

During field-based water quality testing, typically *E. coli* or TTCs are measured because they are good indicators of fecal contamination. Additionally, viral and protozoan testing is difficult outside of a laboratory setting. A variety of field-based tests exist to measure *E. coli* or TTCs. A summary of selected products based on the type of bacterial methods described in the laboratory methods is shown in table 2.4, adapted with permission from Bain et al. (2012). This summary provides information on individual tests. In some cases tests can usefully be combined to cover a range of contamination; for example, Chuang, Trottier, and Murcott (2011) recommended combining Petrifilm™ with a PA test to detect both low (<1 per 100 mL) and high (>100 per 100 mL) levels of *E. coli*.

An often difficult logistical challenge in field-based microbial testing is the requirement to incubate samples. Remote, resource-limited areas may not allow for charging of incubators, or incubators may be too cumbersome to bring along as field equipment. As an alternative, field workers have used phase-change incubators, body temperature, or simply ambient temperature. Brown and Sobsey (2011) found that ambient temperature incubation may be sufficient in some settings; therefore, the use of an incubator should not necessarily be considered a limiting factor when performing field-based microbial testing.

Table 2.4 Catalogue of Presence–Absence and Other Quantitative Microbial Drinking Water Tests

RT	Room temperature	TC	Total coliforms
x	Equipment or resource required	H₂S	Hydrogen sulfide production
Δ	Varies	EC	*Escherichia coli*
?	Value not known	TTC	Thermotolerant coliforms
−	No/poor	S	Small
+	Yes/moderate	M	Medium
++	Good	L	Large
+++	Best	n.a.	Not applicable

Resource settings: Suitable / Not ideal / Not suitable

Type	Product	Cost per test[a]	Cost of specialist equipment[b]	Analysis time (mins.)	Trained technician	Controlled incubation	Ultraviolet light	Sterilization/ disinfection	Deionized water	Cold storage	Transport	Disposal	Sample volume meeting WHO Guideline (100 ml)	Undiluted range (per 100 ml)	Precision	Indicator	Sanitary significance	Standard or approved	Time to result (hrs.)	Shelf-life (mos.)	Temperature (°C)	Low resource	Medium resource	High resource
Presence– absence	**Hydrogen sulfide**																							
	PathoScreen™	$0.60	$0	<5				x				S	−	>5	n.a.	H₂S	+		24–72	12	RT			
	LTEK H₂S 20 ml	$0.80	$0	<5				x				S	−	>5	n.a.	H₂S	+		24–72	24	RT			
	HiWater™	$2.40	$100	<5				x				M	+	>1	n.a.	H₂S	+		24–72	24	RT			
	LTEK H₂S 100 ml	$1.50	$0	<5				x				M	−	>5	n.a.	H₂S	+		24–72	12	RT			
	Local manufacture	Δ	$0	<5				x				S	Δ	Δ	n.a.	H₂S	+		24–72	Δ	RT			
Total coliform	Lamotte® Coliform	$1.20	$0	<5				x				S	−	>10	n.a.	TC	+		44–48	24	RT			
	Rapid HiColiform™	$0.80	$100	<5		x		x			x	M	+	>1	n.a.	TC	+		24	36	2–8			

table continues next page

Table 2.4 Catalogue of Presence–Absence and Other Quantitative Microbial Drinking Water Tests *(continued)*

Type			Product	Cost per test[a]	Cost of specialist equipment[b]	Analysis time (mins.)	Trained technician	Controlled incubation	Ultraviolet light	Sterilization/ disinfection	Deionized water	Cold storage	Transport	Disposal	Sample volume meeting WHO Guideline (100 ml)	Undiluted range (per 100 ml)	Precision	Indicator	Sanitary significance	Standard or approved	Time to result (hrs.)	Shelf-life (mos.)	Temperature (°C)	Low resource	Medium resource	High resource
Presence–absence	E. coli and total coliform		Coliert® 10 ml	$1.50	$100	<5		×	×	×			×	S	–	>10	n.a.	TC&EC	+++	×	24	12	4–30			
			Coliert® 100 ml	$5.00	$100	<5		×	×	×			×	M	+	>1	n.a.	TC&EC	+++	×	24	12	4–30			
			Colisure®	$5.00	$100	<5		×	×	×			×	M	+	>1	n.a.	TC&EC	+++	×	24	12	2–25			
			Coliert® 18	$5.00	$100	<5		×	×	×			×	M	+	>1	n.a.	TC&EC	+++	×	18	15	2–25			
			Modified Colitag™	$4.50	$100	<5		×	×	×			×	M	+	>1	n.a.	TC&EC	+++	×	16	22	4–30			
			Watercheck™ [BWB][c]	$5.00	$2,700	<5		×	×	×			×	M	+	>1	n.a.	TC&EC	+++		24	36	2–30			
			Readycult®	$3.00	$100	<5		×	×	×			×	M	+	>1	n.a.	TC&EC	+++	×	24	36	15–25			
			E*Colite	$3.00	$100	<5		×	×				×	M	+	>1	n.a.	TC&EC	+++	×	28	12	RT			
			EC Blue 100P	$3.70	$100	<5		×	×	×			×	M	+	>1	n.a.	TC&EC	+++		24	12	RT			
			AquaCHROM™	$2.60	$0	<5		×		×			×	M	+	>1	n.a.	TC&EC	+++		18	24	15–30			
			HiSelective™ E. coli	$2.20	$0	<5		×		×			×	M	+	>1	n.a.	TC&EC	+++		24–48	12	2–8			

table continues next page

25

Table 2.4 Catalogue of Presence–Absence and Other Quantitative Microbial Drinking Water Tests *(continued)*

Type	Product	Cost per test[a]	Cost of specialist equipment[b]	Analysis time (mins.)	Trained technician	Controlled incubation	Ultraviolet light	Sterilization/disinfection	Deionized water	Cold storage	Transport	Disposal	Sample volume meeting WHO Guideline (100 ml)	Undiluted range (per 100 ml)	Precision	Indicator	Sanitary significance	Standard or approved	Time to result (hrs.)	Shelf-life (mos.)	Temperature (°C)	Low resource	Medium resource	High resource
Most probable number	**Most probable number**																							
	Compartmentalized bag test	$5–10	$0	<5								S	+	1–43	+	EC	+++		24–72	6–9	RT			
	Coliplate™	$7.50	$200	10	x		x	x		x	x	L	–	5–2,400	+++	TC&EC	+++		24	36	2–30			
	EC BlueQuant	$5.80	$100	5	x		x	x		x	x	L	+	1–1,610	++	TC&EC	+++		24	12	RT			
	Multiple tube (LTB/EC-MUG)	$3.50	$200	30	x	x	x	x	x	x	x	S	Δ	Δ	Δ	EC	+++	x	48	36	RT			
	Multiple tube (LTB/BGLB)	$2.10	$200	30	x	x		x	x		x	S	Δ	Δ	Δ	TC	+	x	36	36	RT			
	Colitag/iMPN1600	$5.77	$0	10	x	x		x		x	x	L	+	1–1,600	++	TC&EC	+++	?	16	22	4–30			
	Colilert/Quanti-Tray®	$5.50	$4,100	10	x	x		x		x	x	L	+	1–200	+++	TC&EC	+++	x	18–24	12	2–25			
	Colilert/Quanti-Tray® 2000	$6.00	$4,100	10	x	x		x		x	x	L	+	1–2,419	+++	TC&EC	+++	x	18–24	12	2–25			
Colony count	**Plate methods**																							
	Petrifilm™ E. coli/Coliform	$1.30	$100	<5	x	x		x		x	x	S	–	100–5,000	+++	TC&EC	+++		24	18	≤8			
	Petrifilm™ Aqua Coliform	$0.70	$100	<5	x	x		x		x	x	S	–	100–5,000	+++	TC	+		24	18	≤8			
	CHROMagar™ ECC	$0.80	$100	15	x	x		x		x	x	S	–	100–5,000	+++	TC&EC	+++		24	36	15–30			
	Compact Dry EC™	$1.00	$0	<5	x	x		x		x	x	S	–	100–5,000	+++	TC&EC	+++		24	24	1–30			

table continues next page

Table 2.4 Catalogue of Presence–Absence and Other Quantitative Microbial Drinking Water Tests (continued)

Type	Product	Cost per test[a]	Cost of specialist equipment[b]	Analysis time (mins.)	Trained technician	Controlled incubation	Ultraviolet light	Sterilization/ disinfection	Deionized water	Cold storage	Transport	Disposal	Sample volume meeting WHO Guideline (100 ml)	Undiluted range (per 100 ml)	Precision	Indicator	Sanitary significance	Standard or approved	Time to result (hrs.)	Shelf-life (mos.)	Temperature (°C)	Low resource	Medium resource	High resource
Colony count																								
Membrane filtration[d]	Portable kit/LSB[e]	$0.50	$2,700	20	x	x		x	x		x	S	△	△	+++	TC&TTC	++		24	48	RT			
	Portable kit/m-coliblue 24™	$2.50	$4,000	15	x	x		x	x		x	M	△	△	+++	TC&TTC	+++	x	24	12	2–8			
	m-Coliblue 24™	$2.50	$2,500	15	x	x		x	x	x	x	M	△	△	+++	TC&EC	+++	x	24	12	2–8			
	Coliscan MF™	$2.20	$2,500	15	x	x		x	x	x	x	M	△	△	+++	TC&EC	+++		24	12	<0			
	m-Endo	$1.50	$2,500	15	x	x		x	x		x	M	△	△	+++	TC	+	x	24	48	RT			
	m-FC	$1.50	$2,500	15	x	x		x	x		x	M	△	△	+++	TTC	++	x	24	48	RT			
	CHROMagar™ Liquid ECC	$1.10	$2,500	15	x	x		x	x		x	M	△	△	+++	TC&EC	+++		24	36	15–30			
	CHROMagar™ ECC	$1.30	$2,500	15	x	x		x	x		x	M	△	△	+++	TC&EC	+++	x	24	36	15–30			
	MI Agar	$1.70	$2,500	15	x	x		x	x		x	M	△	△	+++	TC&EC	+++	x	24	36	RT			
	Chromocult	$1.20	$2,500	15	x	x		x	x		x	M	△	△	+++	TC&EC	+++	x	24	60	RT			
	Rapid E coli	?	$2,500	15	x	x		x	x		x	M	△	△	+++	TC&EC	+++		24	?	?			
Gel based	Coliscan Easygel	$2.20	$0	5	x	x		x		x	x	M	−	20–1,000	+++	TC&EC	+++	x	24	12	<0			
	ColiGel/PathoGel[f]	$3.50	$100	5	x	x	x	x			x	M	+	1–100 (TC) 1–25 (EC)	+++	TC&EC	+++		28	12	RT			

Source: Adapted with permission from Bain et al. 2012.

a. Costs are known to vary greatly from one location to another, depending on supplier, importation taxes, and delivery charges. Where not included in the kit, sample collection vessels are required and add an additional $0.50 per test. For plate methods a disposable pipette at $0.10 has been added.

b. Specific equipment costs are based on: UV torch ($100), membrane filtration assembly, including vacuum pump ($2,500), glassware and racks for multiple tube fermentation ($200), IDEXX Quanti-Tray Sealer ($4,000), and portable membrane filtration kits ($2,700).

c. [BWB] refers to the Bluewater Biosciences Watercheck™ and is not to be confused with the B2P version, denoted [B2P].

d. Costs for membrane filtration are based on three filters.

e. Portable kits are available from a number of manufacturers, including Wagtech, DelAgua, and ELE. The cost varies depending on the kit and ranges from approximately $2,500 to $5,000.

f. PathoGel includes an indicator for H₂S production (PA).

Chemical and Operational Parameters Methods

Most instruments used to measure chemical and operational parameters in the laboratory can also be transferred to the field. Portable versions of spectro-photometers, colorimeters, photometers, pH meters, conductivity meters, and turbidimeters are easily transportable and run on battery storage. Turbidity can also be measured using turbidity tubes, which quantify turbidity by the depth of the water when a mark at the bottom of the tube is no longer visible. Although less accurate than many instruments, it is inexpensive and easily used in the field. Many parameters can be easily measured with color-based test strips that are simply dipped into the sample and read on a color scale. Again, although test strips do not provide an exact measurement, a concentration range is often sufficient for field-testing purposes. Rapid-test kits, such as arsenic test kits, offer the convenience of including all necessary materials to analyze the sample, including reagents and test strips.

Combined Water Quality Laboratories

Portable water quality laboratories can provide several testing methods in one kit. mWater's test kit includes two microbiological tests in order to cover a wider range of detection (PA and colony counting) and additionally includes some chemical parameters, nitrate and chlorine test strips. Hach's CEL Advanced Drinking Water Laboratory[1] includes a colorimeter, multi-meter, several probes, a digital titrator, and reagents, allowing for a variety of chemical tests to be performed. Several products include both microbiological and chemical tests. The DelAgua Testing Kit[2] (photo 2.1a), the Wagtech Potatest[3] (photo 2.1b), and the Trace2o Aquasafe[4] allow for measurement of chemical and physical tests and also include an incubator for membrane filtration–based microbiological testing.

Photo 2.1 Examples of Field Testing Kits

a. DelAgua field kit

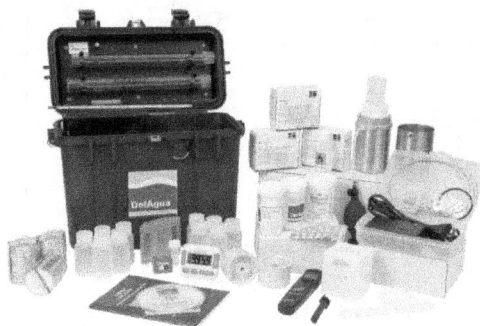

b. Wagtech field kit

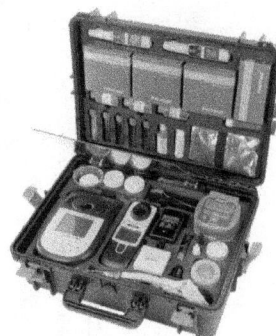

Sources: (a) DelAgua, http://www.delagua.org/delagua-kits; (b) Wagtech, http://www.palintest.com/en/products/wagtech-potatest.

Sanitary Inspections

First introduced in 1991 and published in the WHO monitoring guidelines in 1993, sanitary inspections (SIs) have become a common component of global water quality surveillance programs (Gadgil et al. 1997; Clark et al. 2012; Innovations for Poverty Action 2014). They were developed to provide a rudimentary comparable method for quantifying risk factors that can contribute to microbiological contamination of water sources. SIs include a simple visual assessment of, typically, about 10 risk factor questions, specific to the source type, which are answered with yes or no responses. Each risk factor question is weighted equally (Clasen 2015). The sum of all the "yes" answers is the sanitary inspection score (SIS). The higher the SIS value the higher the category of risk. The SIS and fecal indicator bacteria results can be grouped into risk categories and combined on a risk prioritization matrix (Rice et al. 2012; Innovations for Poverty Action 2014).

In some cases, sanitary surveys have been used to predict microbial contamination, including in guidance provided by WHO, stating,

> It is possible to assess the likelihood of fecal contamination of water sources by a sanitary survey. This is often more valuable than bacteriological testing alone, because a sanitary survey makes it possible to see what needs to be done to protect the water source, and because fecal contamination may vary, so a water sample only represents the quality of the water at the time it was collected (Clark et al. 2012).

However, SIs may have limitations as a method for identifying contaminated drinking water sources. In a recent study, SIs TTC testing among 7,317 unique water sources in West Bengal, India, indicated that the SIS has poor ability to identify TTC-contaminated sources. Aggregating over all source types, the sensitivity (true positive rate) of a high/very high SIS for TTC contamination (TTC > 0 colony forming unit/100 mL) was 29.4 percent and the specificity (true negative rate) was 77.9 percent, resulting in substantial misclassification of the sites when using the established risk categories (Snoad et al. 2017).

Similarly, another recent study in Kenya collected SIs and tested for TTCs. In this study, 100 percent of 20 dug wells, 95 percent of springs, and 61 percent of rainwater systems were contaminated with TTC, with no significant association found between TTC levels and overall sanitary survey scores or individual questions (Misati et al. 2017). These findings suggest some limitations in the use of sanitary surveys as screening tools for identifying TTC contamination at water points.

Notes

1. For more information on Hach, see the company's website, http://www.hach.com/cel-advanced-drinking-water-laboratory/product?id=16602433208.

2. For more information on DelAgua testing kits, see the company's website, http://www.delagua.org/delagua-kits.

3. For more information on the Wagtech Potatest, see Palintest's website, http://www.palintest.com/en/products/wagtech-potatest.

4. For more information on Trace2o Aquasafe testing kits, see the company's website, http://www.trace2o.com/shop/aquasafe-wsl25-pro/.

References

Bain, R., J. Bartram, M. Elliott, R. Matthews, L. McMahan, R. Tung, P. Chuang, and S. Gundry. 2012. "A Summary Catalogue of Microbial Drinking Water Tests for Low and Medium Resource Settings." *International Journal of Environmental Research and Public Health* 9 (5): 1609–25.

Brown, J., and M. Sobsey. 2011. "Evaluating Household Water Treatment Options: Health-Based Targets and Microbiological Performance Specifications." *Water Resources* 68.

Chuang, P., S. Trottier, and S. Murcott. 2011. "Comparison and Verification of Four Field-Based Microbiological Tests: H_2S Test, Easygel®, Colilert®, Petrifilm™." *Journal of Water Sanitation and Hygiene for Development* 1 (1): 68–85.

Clark, P. A., C. A. Pinedo, M. Fadus, and S. Capuzzi. 2012. "Slow-Sand Water Filter: Design, Implementation, Accessibility and Sustainability in Developing Countries." *Medical Science Monitor* 18 (7): RA105–17.

Clasen, T. 2015. "Household Water Treatment and Safe Storage to Prevent Diarrheal Disease in Developing Countries." *Current Environmental Health Reports* 2: 69–74.

EPA (U.S. Environmental Protection Agency). 2001. "Method 1602: Male-specific (F +) and Somatic Coliphage in Water by Single Agar Layer (SAL) Procedure April 2001." EPA Document 821-R-01-029. EPA, Washington, DC.

———. 2005. "Method 1623: Cryptosporidium and Giardia in Water by Filtration/IMS/FA." EPA, Washington, DC.

———. 2016a. "Clean Water Act Analytical Methods." EPA, Washington, DC.

———. 2016b. "Secondary Drinking Water Standards: Guidance for Nuisance Chemicals." EPA, Washington, DC.

Gadgil, A., A. Drescher, D. Greene, P. Miller, C. Motau, and F. Stevens. 1997. "Field Testing UV Disinfection of Drinking Water." 23rd Water, Engineering and Development Centre Conference, Durban, South Africa, September 1–5.

Harwood, V. J., S. Jiang, and M. D. Sobsey. 2015. *Review of Coliphages as Possible Indicator Organisms of Fecal Contamination for Ambient Water Quality*. Washington, DC: EPA.

Innovations for Poverty Action. 2014. "Chlorine Dispensers for Safe Water in Kenya." New Haven, CT.

ISO (International Organization for Standardization). 2016. "Standards Catalogue, 13.060: Water Quality." ISO, Geneva.

Misati, A. G., G. Ogendi, R. Peletz, R. Khush, and E. Kumpel. 2017. "Can Sanitary Surveys Replace Water Quality Testing? Evidence from Kisii, Kenya." *International Journal of Environmental Research and Public Health* 14 (2): 152.

Rice, E. W., R. B. Baird, A. D. Eaton, and L. S. Clesceri. 2012. *Standard Methods for the Examination of Water and Wastewater*. 22nd ed. Washington, DC: American Water Works Association.

Snoad, C., C. Nagel, A. Bhattacharya, and E. Thomas. 2017. "The Effectiveness of Sanitary Inspections as a Risk Assessment Tool for Thermotolerant Coliform Bacteria Contamination of Rural Drinking Water: A Review of Data from West Bengal, India." *The American Journal of Tropical Medicine and Hygiene* 96 (4): 976–83.

WHO (World Health Organization). 2011a. *Evaluating Household Water Treatment Options: Health-Based Targets and Microbiological Performance Specifications*. Geneva: WHO.

———. 2011b. *Guidelines for Drinking-Water Quality*. Geneva: WHO.

———. 2012. *Chemical Safety of Drinking-Water: Assessing Priorities for Risk Management*. Geneva: WHO.

CHAPTER 3

Sanitation and Hygiene Monitoring

Nick Turman-Bryant

Introduction

An inherent challenge in monitoring sanitation programs is the diversity of behaviors and facilities. Sanitation behaviors encompass defecation, urination, anal cleansing, deposition of children's feces, deposition of cleansing products, separation of solid and liquid waste, fecal sludge management, handwashing, adherence to sanitation facility use, and menstrual hygiene. There are also many types of sanitation facilities that separate excreta from human contact with varying degrees of efficacy (for example, open defecation versus a flush toilet connected to a sewer system). Finally, there are additional factors that can influence the level of contamination in a sanitation facility, including the latrine's cleanliness, whether it is shared or private, and the degree to which all members of a household can access it. These layers of behavior, facility type, and facility characteristics interact dynamically and change in time, making it difficult to determine which sanitation features are most important for reducing human exposure to pathogens. Given this complexity, it is important to identify the sanitation outcomes that minimize exposure to pathogens before exploring the best practices and technologies for monitoring those outcomes.

This chapter identifies outcomes that are explicitly or implicitly identified in the Sustainable Development Goal (SDG) target on sanitation and hygiene and the extent to which those outcomes are represented in the proposed service ladders. A variety of innovative practices and technologies are described with specific attention given to their abilities to accurately measure and monitor progress on each outcome.

Sanitation Outcomes

SDG target 6.2 states, "By 2030, achieve access to adequate and equitable sanitation and hygiene for all and end open defecation, paying special attention to the needs of women and girls and those in vulnerable situations" (WHO/UNICEF 2015, 4). Whereas the Millennium Development Goal (MDG) target emphasized a single outcome—access to improved sanitation facilities—the SDG

Figure 3.1 Aspects of Access and the Scales on Which They Apply

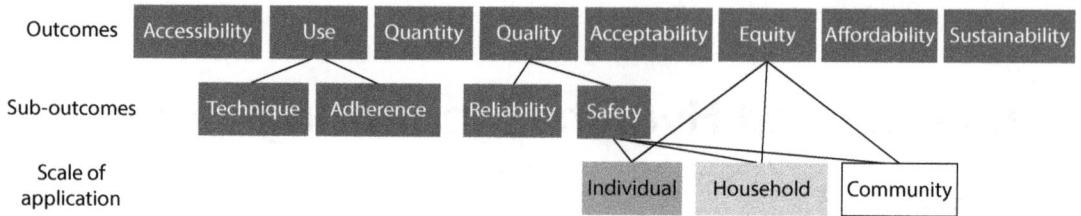

sanitation target builds on this by incorporating adequacy and equity. This expanded understanding of access acknowledges that structural and relational mechanisms also influence an individual's ability to derive benefits from sanitation services (Ribot and Peluso 2003). An amplified definition of access that moves beyond coverage is depicted in figure 3.1.

Sanitation Ladder

Recognizing that sanitation services can include a variety of levels, the Joint Monitoring Programme (JMP) has updated its service ladder to define five thresholds of service. Like the service ladder used for the MDG sanitation target, three of the categories designate the type of sanitation facility: unimproved, limited, or basic. Figure 3.2 maps these categories from the proposed sanitation ladder to the outcomes expressed implicitly or explicitly in target 6.2. In the figure, "open defecation" describes the deposition of human feces directly in the environment, and "safely managed" designates a basic sanitation facility that is not shared and where excreta are safely disposed in situ or treated off-site.

- **Accessibility:** Accessibility is defined as "facilities that are close to home that can be easily reached and used when needed" (WHO/UNICEF 2015, 11). Accessibility is well represented in the proposed service ladder, with access being inferred directly from the sanitation facility type and whether it is shared. Although accessibility can change in time because of changes in the functionality of the sanitation facility or how much it is being shared, this outcome has the strongest representation in the ladder.

- **Household safety:** The safety of the sanitation facility for the household—how well it separates excreta from human contact within the household—is not represented in the ladder. Household safety is indirectly inferred from the sanitation facility type, where basic sanitation facilities are assumed to adequately separate excreta from household contact and unimproved sanitation facilities are not.

Figure 3.2 Mapping the Proposed Sanitation Ladder to the Desired Outcomes

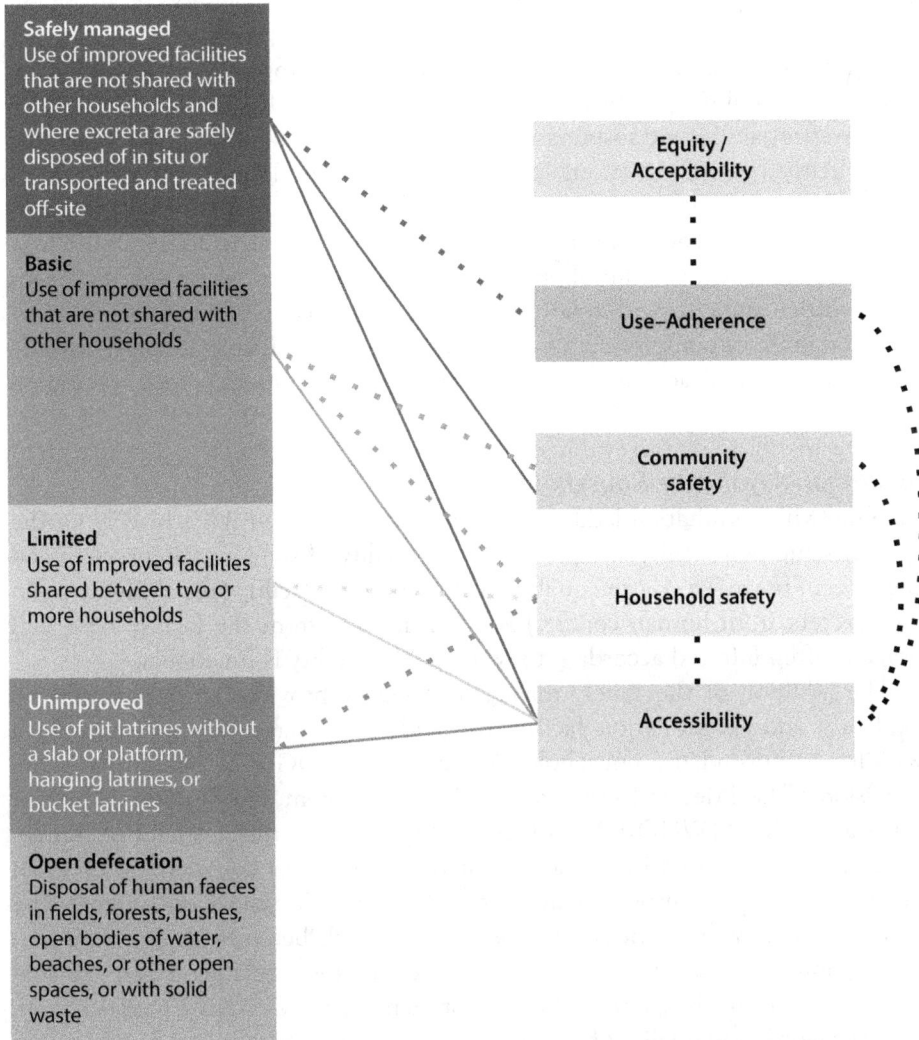

Source: Adapted from the new JMP ladder for sanitation services, WHO/UNICEF 2017.
Note: Improved facilities include flush/pour flush to piped sewer systems, septic tanks, or pit latrines; ventilated improved pit latrines; composting toilets; or pit latrines with slabs.

- **Community safety:** The safety of the sanitation facility for the community—how well it separates excreta from human contact beyond the household—is better represented in the ladder. Like household safety, community safety is inferred indirectly from the sanitation facility type, but community safety is addressed directly by the "safely managed" category. There is a broad and growing recognition that sanitation services must be applied on multiple scales to be effective, and the addition of the "safely managed" category to the service ladder provides the first indicator of how fecal waste is managed beyond the household.

- **Use–Adherence:** Although sanitation facility use is key for realizing health benefits, adherence is not addressed explicitly in any of the service categories.

- **Equity/Acceptability:** Equity is defined as the "progressive reduction and elimination of inequalities between sub-groups" (WHO/UNICEF 2015, 11). Like affordability and sustainability, equity and acceptability are not addressed explicitly by the sanitation ladder. Although population-level inequalities could be inferred from adoption rates or the elimination of inequalities across population subgroups, more direct measures of equity and acceptability may be needed to capture intrahousehold inequalities (that is, the specific needs of women and girls within households) and the acceptability of specific sanitation interventions. If reliable measures of use are available, it is also possible that equity and acceptability could be inferred indirectly from sanitation facility use.

Sanitation beyond the Household

Like the MDG sanitation ladder, the new sanitation ladder relies heavily on the type of sanitation facility as a proxy for the quality of the sanitation service and the level of usage. That is, the quality of the sanitation facility (the ability to separate excreta from human contact) is often inferred from the facility type, and usage is often inferred according to whether the facility is functional.

The addition of the "safely managed" category provides an opportunity to explicitly address sanitation facility use and how excreta are managed both within and beyond the household. As defined in SDG 6.2, "Sanitation is the provision of facilities and services for safe management and disposal of human urine and faeces" (WHO/UNICEF 2015, 11). The safe management of human waste comprises an entire service chain that starts with containment and can include collection, transport, treatment, and reuse or disposal. Consequently, the quality of sanitation services must be distinguished "between those relating to safe separation of excreta from human contact and those relating to safe removal of excreta from the household environment" (WHO/UNICEF 2015, 19). In other words, the quality of a sanitation service must be evaluated with regard to household safety as well as community safety. Although the improved/unimproved designation under the MDGs provided insight into the quality of sanitation for the household, it shed little light on how excreta were being managed beyond the household. In contrast, the "safely managed" category explicitly addresses the quality of the sanitation facility for the community by stating that excreta must be safely disposed in situ or treated off-site.

Sanitation Indicators

Although the inclusion of the "safely managed" category represents substantial progress in the evolution of the service ladder, there is still a great deal of ambiguity surrounding the indicators that will be used to monitor outcomes. Currently, the JMP plans to use household surveys and regulatory data as the main data source for observing household sanitation facility types. The sanitation facility type and attributes will then be used to infer other outcomes like safety and use. For example, lack of use could be inferred directly from a nonfunctioning toilet, and unimproved sanitation facilities would be assumed to provide unsafe management both within and beyond the household (WHO/UNICEF 2015, 27).

The JMP indicators also acknowledge that monitoring the safe management of excreta requires a full fecal waste flow framework that spans the service chain from containment to reuse or disposal. Although information about containment can be collected from household surveys, the JMP proposes to monitor the emptying, transport, and treatment of fecal waste using a combination of utility, population, and household data to estimate safe management through the service chain. As a result, "reuse and disposal would not be monitored initially at a global level" (WHO/UNICEF 2015, 28). On-site treatment and disposal would be inferred according to a variety of factors, including the sanitation facility type, construction quality, frequency of use, population density, geographic conditions, and urban versus rural location (WHO/UNICEF 2015). Off-site treatment will initially be estimated from utility records according to the number of sewer connections and installed treatment facilities. Off-site treatment for excreta that are collected and transported from septic tanks and pit latrines could then be estimated using records from trucks disposing waste at wastewater treatment plants (WHO/UNICEF 2015).

Monitoring Sanitation Outcomes

The following section provides an overview of relevant practices and technologies for monitoring sanitation outcomes. Because no one practice or technology is adequate for monitoring progress in sanitation, it is important to note that some practices and technologies are better suited for monitoring specific sanitation outcomes. Figure 3.3 provides a visual mapping of each methodology to each sanitation outcome.

Accessibility

Household surveys and national censuses are the most common methodologies used for assessing a household's access to sanitation facilities (Clasen et al. 2012). There are various advantages to using surveys for evaluating access. First, as two of the most common tools for gathering household information, surveys and censuses provide a growing knowledge base that facilitates comparison across time and geography. Second, appropriate survey design can result in higher validity and reliability of survey responses. Third, administering surveys in households allows for interaction with household members and direct observation of sanitation facilities. Thus, although survey questions can differentiate which members of the household are able to access a sanitation facility, direct observation allows an observer to verify the sanitation facility type, its functionality, whether it is

Figure 3.3 Monitoring Methodologies and Technologies for Sanitation Outcomes

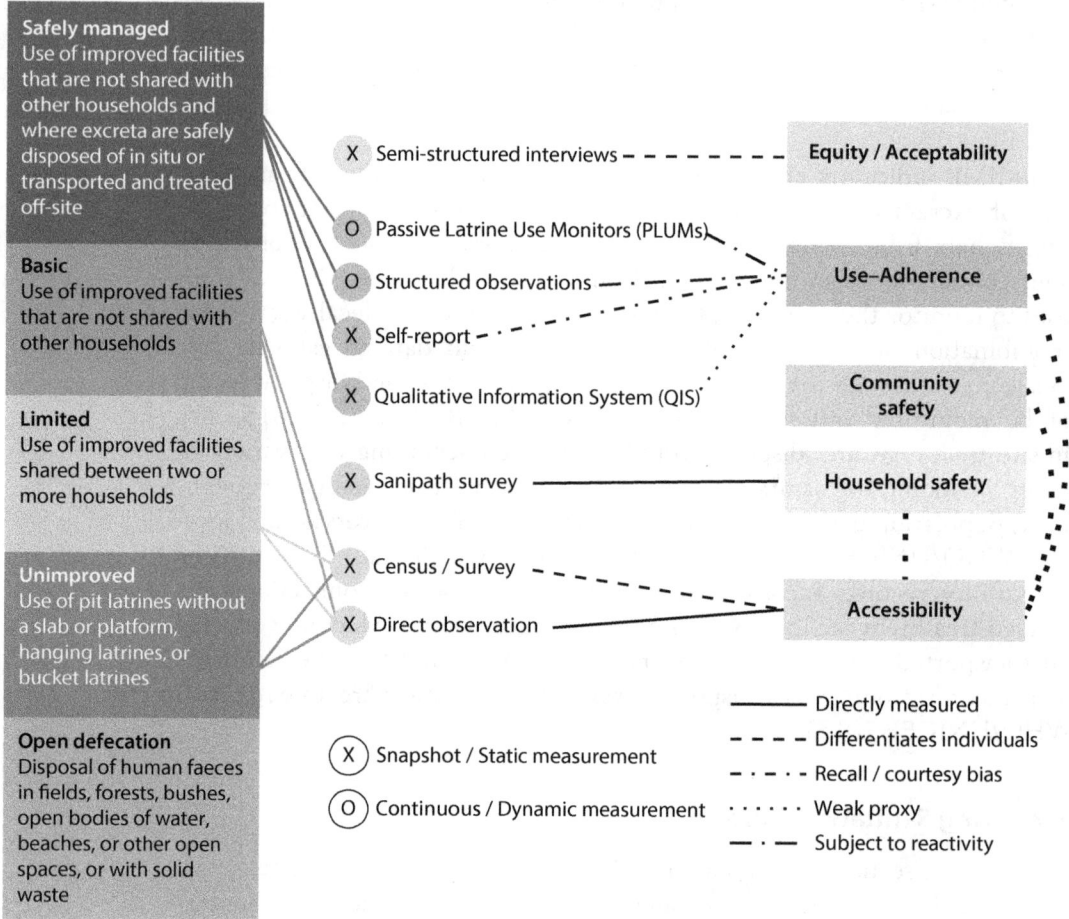

Source: Adapted from the new JMP ladder for sanitation services, WHO/UNICEF 2017.
Note: Improved facilities include flush/pour flush to piped sewer systems, septic tanks, or pit latrines; ventilated improved pit latrines; composting toilets; or pit latrines with slabs.

private or shared, and its proximity to the household. Still, unless there are repeated visits to the household, census surveys and spot checks provide only a static measurement of the sanitation facility's accessibility and functionality (Thomas and Mattson 2013).

Household Safety

The type of sanitation facility and whether it is private are the two main prox-ies used to determine whether excreta are safely separated from human contact within the household. However, there are very few methods for directly measuring the quality of specific sanitation facilities. One exception is the Sanipath Rapid Assessment Tool created by researchers at the Center for Global Safe Water at Emory University. The Sanipath tool provides an assessment of exposure to fecal contamination by measuring the level of fecal contamination associated with different transmission pathways (such as drinking water, latrines, produce, open drains, and so on). These microbial loads are combined with surveys that characterize household behaviors to generate risk assessments for each exposure pathway. For example, a household may use a private pit latrine with a slab, but the Sanipath tool could be used to estimate the actual risk of exposure to fecal contaminants according to the level of contamination in the latrine and the behaviors of the users. Although the Sanipath tool is primarily designed to evaluate the level of exposure to fecal contamination for an entire community, the methodology could be adapted to the household scale. The ability to combine microbial testing with survey responses is also a strength because the surveys facilitate a more nuanced characterization of individual sanitation and hygiene practices. However, the tool depends on the ability of local laboratories to conduct testing in a sterile environment with sufficient equipment. Also, unless the Sanipath assessment is performed regularly, the measurement represents a one-time snapshot that does not monitor changes in behavior, fecal contamination in the environment, or the functionality of sanitation facilities.[1]

Community Safety

Very few methodologies have been developed to directly verify the safe management of excreta beyond the household. Although safe management is often assumed for sanitation facilities that are connected to a sewer system, septic tank, or pit latrine, the actual verification of waste removal, transport, and treatment represents a significant challenge for monitoring community safety. Data from utilities could be used to estimate the safe treatment of excreta on the basis of the number of household connections and the conveyance to installed treatment facilities. Similarly, records from disposal trucks could be used to estimate the number of households from which waste is safely collected and removed. However, unless records from the point of collection to the point of treatment can be corroborated, utility and waste removal estimates may underestimate leakage or the deposition of waste directly into the environment.

Although they may not provide an accurate measure of the level of exposure to fecal contamination in the environment, records from utilities and waste collectors can be used to verify that excreta are being collected and conveyed to treatment facilities. For example, Sanergy Inc. in Kenya has partnered with SweetSense Inc. to use motion sensors to optimize sanitation waste collection operations. The sensors are also able to send alerts from the latrine operator or the waste collector through radio frequency identification tags that are directly integrated into Salesforce. Similarly, x-runner in Peru and the Water and Sanitation Program in India are able to track the installation and management of improved toilets through near-field communication tags and barcodes that are scanned and tracked through Salesforce and Open Data Kit (Robiarto et al. 2014; Nique and Smertnik 2015).

Use–Adherence

Although not explicitly represented in the sanitation ladder, sanitation facility use and adherence are key indicators for measuring sanitation facility efficacy (Clasen et al. 2014). However, the verification of sanitation facility use and a household's adherence to use is incredibly challenging.

Clasen et al. (2012, 3296) suggest that spot-check indicators and sanitary surveys "are subjective and may lack necessary sensitivity and specificity to quantify patterns of use." In an experiment comparing latrine use recorded by motion detector sensors or structured observations, they found that sensor-recorded use and observed use agreed within two latrine use events 93.9 percent of the time over 228 observation periods. They also found strong evidence of reactivity to structured observation because the sensors recorded significantly more latrine events during observation periods compared to non-observation periods (Clasen et al. 2012). O'Reilly et al. (2015) also recorded a high level of agreement between sensor-reported events and structured observations.

In a similar study, Sinha et al. (2016) found that mean reported "usual" daily use was almost twice the average daily sensor-recorded use (7.09 versus 3.62 events). Although there was better agreement between reported use and sensor-recorded use from the previous 48 hours (4.61 versus 3.59 events), the predicted number of latrine events using the 48-hour recall measure was still 60 percent greater than the average number of events recorded by the sensors. See chapter 5 for additional technical descriptions of these latrine sensors.

BRAC in Bangladesh has developed a Qualitative Information System (QIS) that incorporates a combination of spot-check indicators with survey questions to assess latrine use. In a study comparing three latrine use measurement methodologies including surveys, observations, and motion detector sensors, there was a strong correlation between latrine spot-check indicators and BRAC's QIS indicators. There was also a positive correlation between self-reported latrine use and sensor-recorded latrine use, although self-reported use was significantly greater than sensor-recorded use. Although households reported an average of 32.8 latrine uses over four days, sensors recorded an average of 21.7 uses, perhaps indicating recall or courtesy bias in self-reporting (Delea 2015). Given the different scales used, no comparison was drawn between sensor-recorded use or self-reported use and the spot-check indicators.

Equity/Acceptability

Although elimination of inequalities and the special needs of women and girls are addressed in the sanitation target, the JMP's current proposal for measuring inequalities involves a comparison of population subgroups that are disaggregated by "income, gender, age, race, ethnicity, migratory status, disability, geographic location, and other characteristics relevant in national contexts" (WHO/UNICEF 2015, 17). However, evidence shows that inequalities in sanitation facility use can occur on an intrahousehold scale as well as on a societal scale (Jenkins and Curtis 2005; Gupta et al. 2014). In addition, more nuanced methodologies may be necessary to incorporate the specific needs of women and girls to ensure the acceptability, security, and privacy of sanitation facilities. Given the sensitivity of sanitation subjects and the influences of cultural and religious norms, qualitative methodologies like ethnography and semistructured interviews may be needed to accurately gauge acceptability and characterize intra-household sanitation behaviors. For example, O'Reilly et al. (2015) found that ethnographic and motion detector data were highly complementary and useful for comparing sanitation practices between groups that differed in geography and religious affinity.

Hygiene Outcomes and the Service Ladder

Given that hygiene was not addressed in the MDG targets, its inclusion in SDG 6.2 highlights the growing consensus that water, sanitation, and hygiene (WASH) are indelibly linked and cannot be treated in isolation. Hygiene is defined as "the conditions and practices that help maintain health and prevent disease including handwashing, menstrual hygiene management and food hygiene" (WHO/UNICEF 2015, 20). Although food hygiene was identified as one of the top priorities for health and nutrition, it was ultimately determined to be outside the scope of WASH monitoring. Similarly, menstrual hygiene management is mentioned but is not addressed specifically in the indicators. Thus, hygiene as described by the service ladder is primarily concerned with handwashing. Like sanitation, adequate and equitable access to hygiene involves accessibility, use, and equity/acceptability. Unlike sanitation, the quality of the service depends more on the practice of the individual—handwashing efficacy—than the function of the facility.

As seen in figure 3.4, the proposed handwashing ladder designates three thresholds of hygiene service: no handwashing facility, a limited handwashing facility without soap or without water, and a basic handwashing facility with soap and water. Similar to the sanitation ladder, it is worth exploring how well the handwashing ladder matches up with the desired outcomes.

- **Accessibility:** Accessibility is well represented again, with access being inferred directly from the handwashing facility and whether soap and water are present.
- **Use–Technique:** The ability to remove contamination from the hands depends a great deal on how effectively the hands are washed and whether soap is used. Although none of the service categories addresses handwashing technique, it still figures prominently in determining the effectiveness of hygiene interventions.
- **Use–Adherence:** Regular handwashing that coincides with sanitation behaviors is also important for realizing health benefits. Although not addressed directly in the service ladder, handwashing practice is often inferred indirectly from the presence of handwashing facilities.
- **Equity/Acceptability:** Equity and acceptability can also be indirectly inferred from regular use by all members of the household, but more direct measures of equity and acceptability may be needed to ensure that the specific needs of women and girls are being met, particularly regarding menstrual hygiene management.

Figure 3.4 Mapping the Proposed Handwashing Ladder to the Desired Outcomes

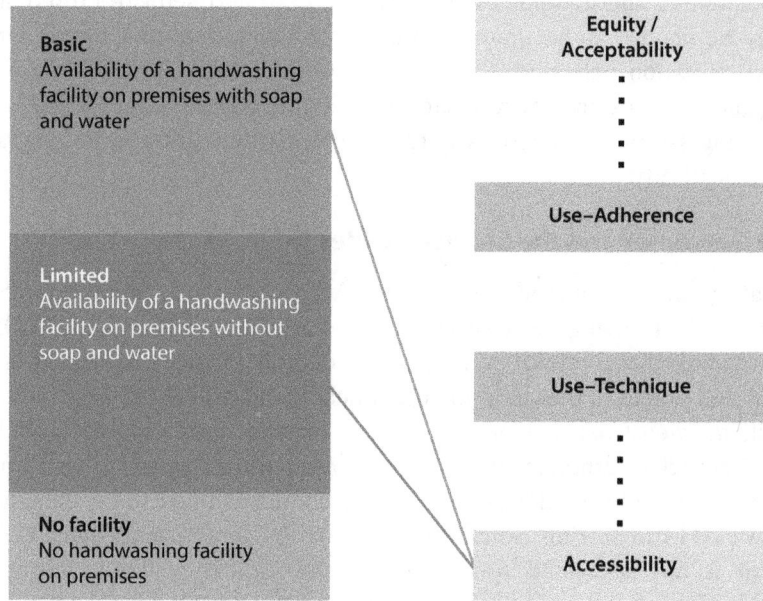

Source: Adapted from the new JMP ladder for hygiene, WHO/UNICEF 2017.

Like the sanitation ladder, the handwashing ladder uses the presence of a handwashing facility as a proxy for use. Equity, acceptability, and handwashing efficacy are not explicitly addressed in the proposed handwashing ladder.

Monitoring Hygiene Outcomes

In contrast to the challenges associated with monitoring progress on sanitation outcomes, the proposed methodology for monitoring progress on hygiene is relatively direct. Since 2009, the JMP has used the "observation of the place where household members wash their hands and the presence of water and soap" as the primary indicators of handwashing behavior (WHO/UNICEF 2015, 21). As a result, the JMP is able to measure the handwashing ladder directly through household surveys and extrapolate those estimates to the broader population base.

Although the monitoring of hygiene facilities is relatively straightforward, the following section provides a summary of different practices and technologies that have been used to monitor hygiene outcomes. Actual handwashing behavior is still challenging to monitor, but it is possible that the type of hygiene facility could serve as an adequate proxy for access and use for mixed-purpose, large population surveys (Ram 2013). Figure 3.5 provides a visual mapping of each methodology to each hygiene outcome.

Figure 3.5 Monitoring Methodologies and Technologies for Hygiene Outcomes

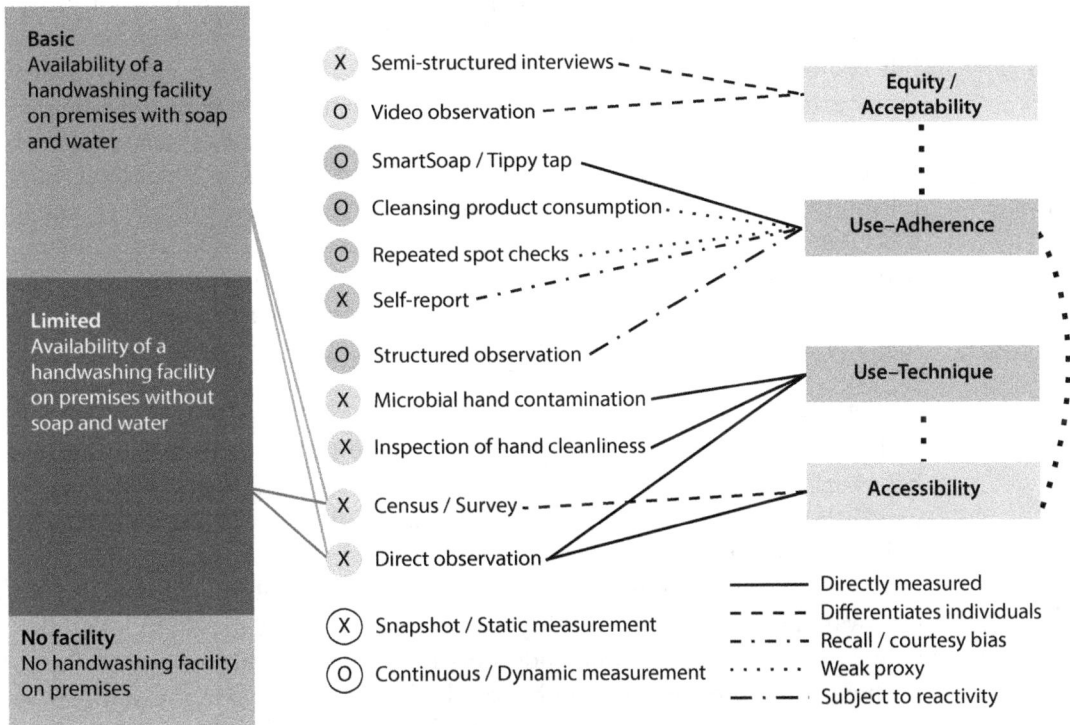

Source: Adapted from the new JMP ladder for hygiene, WHO/UNICEF 2017.

Accessibility

As with sanitation, household surveys and censuses are the easiest indicators for evaluating access to hygiene facilities. Easily combined with spot-check indicators that facilitate direct observation of handwashing facilities and materials, rapid observations are used almost exclusively in large population surveys where hygiene is one among many behaviors of interest. As a direct measure, rapid observations are cost-effective, efficient, and more reliable than survey responses (Cairncross et al. 2005; Ram 2013). However, verification of the handwashing facility does not provide information about individual hygiene practices within the household, whether handwashing is performed at critical times (for example, after defecation or before meals), or the efficacy of handwashing and its consistency across time.

Use–Technique

Measurement of microbial hand contamination through laboratory measurements or visual inspection are two methodologies that are used to verify handwashing efficacy. Although research has shown a positive correlation between hand contamination and health outcomes (Luby et al. 2009; Pickering et al. 2010), measurement of hand contamination is relatively expensive and time-consuming, and may require access to a microbial laboratory facility (Ram 2013). Observation of handwashing practice can be a useful method for verifying the use of soap, the duration of handwashing, and the method for drying; but respondent behavior may be influenced by the presence of an observer (Sagerman et al. 2011). Visual inspections of hand contamination can be performed efficiently and are positively associated with microbial contamination and observed handwashing (Pickering et al. 2010). However, a high inter-rater reliability is important for avoiding subjectivity bias between multiple enumerators (Ram 2013). Also, as a static indicator, the measurement of hand contamination cannot capture how quickly recontamination occurs after washing. For example, Ram et al. (2011) found a high level of recontamination within two hours of a thorough handwashing with soap.

Use–Adherence

Although handwashing with soap at critical times (such as after defecation and before meals) has been identified as one of the most cost-effective behaviors for preventing infection, verification of handwashing adherence remains a challenge. Indicators like the presence of soap and water and handwashing efficacy are positively correlated, but it is still unclear how well these indicators predict handwashing behavior (Ram 2013). For example, Biran et al. (2008) found that only 2 out of 26 handwashing indicators used to classify households as "handwashing"—the presence of soap beside the latrine and soap in the yard—were significantly correlated with classifications of households based on structured observations.

Self-reported behavior is one of the most common indicators used to assess hygienic practice. However, self-reported handwashing usually overestimates actual handwashing because of the social desirability associated with handwashing. For example, although 77 percent of respondents in a Bangladesh study reported handwashing with soap after defecation, only 32 percent were observed to do so (ICDDR,B 2008). When accounting for actual soap use, the discrepancy between reported and observed handwashing persists but decreases slightly (Ram 2013).

Structured observation has typically been used as the gold standard for comparing different handwashing measures. Structured observations can record more detailed information about how hands are washed, when hands are washed, and who washes their hands; but it is important that the timing and location of observations include as many members of the household as possible and critical events like meal preparation and consumption (Biran et al. 2008). Given that an observer's presence has been shown to increase the number of handwashing events by as much as 35 percent, Ram et al. (2010) question whether structured observations should be the standard for comparison because of high reactivity. Unlike self-reports, however, structured observation provides a more dynamic measure of handwashing behavior over time.

Repeated spot checks also provide a more dynamic measure of handwashing behavior. Webb et al. (2006) determined that six separate spot checks are needed to reliably estimate a household's hygiene practices, although repeated visits may also increase reactivity (Arnold et al. 2015).

Although studies that monitor the consumption of cleansing products have been conducted in high-income countries, only a few studies have tracked soap purchases or soap weight differences as a proxy for handwashing behavior (Ram 2013). For example, Gadgil et al. (2011) found a positive correlation between consumption of bar soap and observed handwashing events. However, Luby et al. (2009) observed no differences in soap purchases between the treatment and control groups in a handwashing intervention, despite differences between the two groups in the presence of soap and water and handwashing techniques.

Other methodologies, such as sensors and video observation, have been used to monitor latrine use as well as handwashing behavior. Sensor technologies and applications are reviewed in chapter 5. Video observation also can be an effective tool for observing and recording handwashing behavior unobtrusively. Although no comparisons have been conducted, it is possible that video observation would be preferable to direct observation in settings where handwashing behavior can be clearly recorded from a fixed location. Video observation has the advantage of being able to record over longer periods without interruption, and recordings can be reviewed rapidly by a human observer. It is also possible that discreetly placed video observation may reduce reactivity, although there are ethical concerns that must be considered when consent cannot be obtained for all involved parties. Like sensors, video observation provides a dynamic measure of handwashing behavior over time, but it also allows the reviewer to differentiate the handwashing behaviors of specific individuals (Pickering et al. 2014).

Equity/Acceptability

The goals of equity and acceptability in hygiene practices may require more qualitative methodologies like ethnography and semistructured interviews to understand what motivates hygienic behavior, to gauge the acceptability of hygiene interventions, and to characterize intrahousehold hygiene behaviors. This is particularly true for the special needs of women and girls and the ambiguity surrounding indicators for menstrual hygiene management. For example, Curtis, Danquah, and Aunger (2009) found that social affiliation and disgust were two strong motivators of handwashing behavior but that fear of disease had little influence.

As proposed by Ram (2013), composite measures would ideally be employed to more accurately characterize handwashing behaviors. Although some methodologies are particularly suited to measuring specific outcomes (for example, sensors for monitoring handwashing practices), no one methodology is adequate for verifying and monitoring all four hygiene outcomes.

Indicator Selection

In a recent systematic review of indicator selection methods for WASH monitoring, Schwemlein, Cronk, and Bartram (2016) note a general lack of consistency, specificity, and relevancy in the indicators used by the projects and programs included in their review. In particular, they suggest that better coordination of WASH indicators could help "identify weaknesses in data collection," "inform decisions in WASH policy and practice," and "facilitate comparison of projects, programs, and interventions" (Schwemlein, Cronk, and Bartram 2016, 2). However, they argue that a more formal process for selecting indicators and organizing data collection is needed to improve transparency and improve coordination in WASH interventions.

On the basis of the frequency of indicator selection methods encountered in their review, they propose a six-step method for selecting WASH indicators (see figure 3.6). Notably, they recommend that the indicator selection process should be explicitly tied to the outcomes of interest according to the purpose and scope of the intervention. In addition, they provide three examples of conceptual frameworks that could be used for organizing indicators and facilitating comparison across studies. These include the Driving forces-Pressures-State-Impact-Response, the Social-Economic-Ecologic/Environment, and the Inputs-Outputs-Outcomes-Impacts frameworks. In addition, they suggest that proposed indicators should be evaluated using objective selection criteria, including whether the proposed indicator is measureable, reliable, and sensitive to changes in the outcome of interest. Finally, they argue that candidate indicators must be valid, that is, "[t]here must be an accurate correlation between an indicator and the issue for which it is supposed to proxy" based on existing data (Schwemlein, Cronk, and Bartram 2016, 11).

Figure 3.6 Proposed Method for Indicator Selection for WASH Monitoring

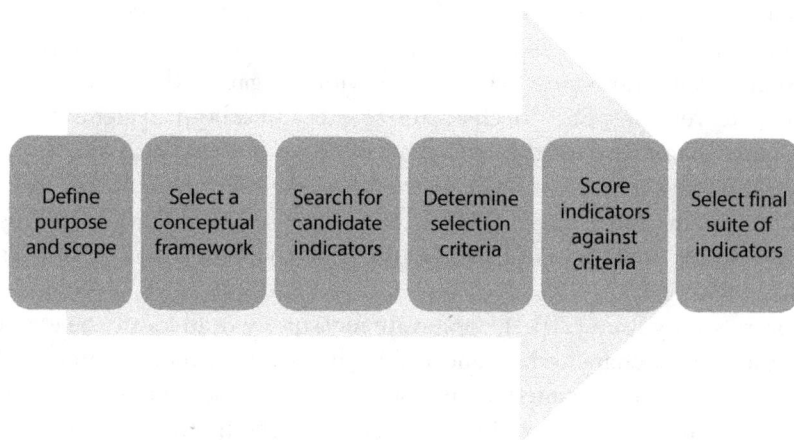

Define purpose and scope → Select a conceptual framework → Search for candidate indicators → Determine selection criteria → Score indicators against criteria → Select final suite of indicators

Source: Schwemlein, Cronk, and Bartram 2016.
Note: WASH = water, sanitation, and hygiene.

Conclusion

Making progress on sanitation and hygiene requires an integrated approach. Health benefits from improved sanitation and hygiene facilities depend on their accessibility, their usage, and their safety for the household and the community. Moreover, attending to the special needs of women and girls will require indicators that are more sensitive to questions of equity and acceptability on a household level as well as a societal level. Finally, given the significant overlap of water, sanitation, hygiene, and nutrition, interventions must be coordinated in an integrated fashion for significant health impacts to be realized.

Although the SDG target for sanitation and hygiene represents a marked improvement over the MDG target, there is still a substantial disconnect between the desired outcomes and the proposed indicators. The inclusion of safety, adequacy, and equity acknowledges that progress cannot be measured by simply counting the number of latrines or soap bars. However, the proposed service ladders still rely heavily on the direct observation of sanitation and handwashing facilities to infer usage and the management of excreta.

Note

1. Information in this section comes from the draft "Rapid Assessment Tool Manual" (accessed December 1, 2015) from sanipath.org.

References

Arnold, B. F., R. S. Khush, P. Ramaswamy, P. Rajkumar, N. Durairaj, P. Ramaprabha, K. Balakrishnan, and J. M. Colford. 2015. "Short Report: Reactivity in Rapidly Collected Hygiene and Toilet Spot Check Measurements: A Cautionary Note for Longitudinal Studies." *American Journal of Tropical Medicine and Hygiene* 92 (1): 159–62.

Biran, A., T. Rabie, W. Schmidt, S. Juvekar, S. Hirve, and V. Curtis. 2008. "Comparing the Performance of Indicators of Hand-Washing Practices in Rural Indian Households." *Tropical Medicine and International Health* 13 (2): 278–85.

Cairncross, S., K. Shordt, S. Zacharia, and B. K. Govindan. 2005. "What Causes Sustainable Changes in Hygiene Behaviour? A Cross-Sectional Study from Kerala, India." *Social Science and Medicine* 61 (10): 2212–20.

Clasen, T., S. Boisson, P. Routray, B. Torondel, M. Bell, O. Cumming, J. Ensink, M. Freeman, M. Jenkins, M. Odagiri, S. Ray, A. Sinha, M. Suar, and W.-P. Schmidt. 2014. "Effectiveness of a Rural Sanitation Programme on Diarrhoea, Soil-Transmitted Helminth Infection, and Child Malnutrition in Odisha, India: A Cluster-Randomised Trial." *The Lancet Global Health* 2 (11): e645–53.

Clasen, T., D. Fabini, S. Boisson, J. Taneja, J. Song, E. Aichinger, A. Bui, S. Dadashi, W. P. Schmidt, Z. Burt, and K. L. Nelson. 2012. "Making Sanitation Count: Developing and Testing a Device For Assessing Latrine Use in Low-Income Settings." *Environmental Science and Technology* 46 (6): 3295–303.

Curtis, V. A., L. O. Danquah, and R. V. Aunger. 2009. "Planned, Motivated and Habitual Hygiene Behaviour: An Eleven Country Review." *Health Education Research* 24 (4): 655–73.

Delea, M. 2015. "Report on a Study to Independently Assess Latrine Coverage and Use under BRAC's WASH II Project in Bangladesh." Internal report submitted to Gates Foundation.

Gadgil, M. A., L. Unicomb, S. P. Luby, and P. K. Ram. 2011. "Consistent Soap Availability Correlates with Use of Inexpensive Soap Products and Improved Handwashing in Low-Income Households in Dhaka, Bangladesh." Presented at the American Society of Tropical Medicine and Hygiene Annual Meeting, Philadelphia, PA, December 4–8.

Gupta A., D. Spears, D. Coffey, N. Khurana, N. Srivastav, P. Hathi, and S. Vyas. 2014. "Revealed Preference for Open Defecation." *Economic and Political Weekly* 49 (38): 43–55.

ICDDR,B (International Centre for Diarrhoeal Disease Research, Bangladesh). 2008. "Handwashing Behavior in Rural Bangladesh." *Health and Science Bulletin* 6 (3).

Jenkins, M. W., and V. Curtis. 2005. "Achieving the 'Good Life': Why Some People Want Latrines in Rural Benin." *Social Science and Medicine* 61 (11): 2446–59.

Luby, S. P., A. K. Halder, C. Tronchet, S. Akhter, A. Bhuiya, and R. B. Johnston. 2009. "Household Characteristics Associated with Handwashing with Soap in Rural Bangladesh." *The American Journal of Tropical Medicine and Hygiene* 81(5): 882–87.

Nique, M., and H. Smertnik. 2015. "The Role of Mobile in Improved Sanitation Access." GSMA Mobile for Development Utilities Programme. https://www.gsma.com/mobi lefordevelopment/wp-content/uploads/2015/08/The-Role-of-Mobile-in-Improved -Sanitation-Access.pdf.

O'Reilly, K., E. Louis, E. Thomas, and A. Sinha. 2015. "Combining Sensor Monitoring and Ethnography to Evaluate Household Latrine Usage in Rural India." *Journal of Water, Sanitation and Hygiene for Development* 5 (3): 426.

Pickering, A. J., A. G. Blum, R. F. Breiman, P. K. Ram, and J. Davis. 2014. "Video Surveillance Captures Student Hand Hygiene Behavior, Reactivity to Observation, and Peer Influence in Kenyan Primary Schools." *PLoS ONE* 9 (3): 1–7.

Pickering, A. J., A. B. Boehm, M. Mwanjali, and J. Davis. 2010. "Efficacy of Waterless Hand Hygiene Compared with Handwashing with Soap: A Field Study in Dar es Salaam, Tanzania." *The American Journal of Tropical Medicine and Hygiene* 82 (2): 270–78.

Ram, P. 2013. "Practical Guidance for Measuring Handwashing Behavior: 2013 Update." Water and Sanitation Working Paper, World Bank, Washington, DC.

Ram, P. K., A. K. Halder, S. P. Granger, T. Jones, P. Hall, D. Hitchcock, R. Wright, B. Nygren, M. S. Islam, J. W. Molyneaux, and S. P. Luby. 2010. "Is Structured Observation a Valid Technique to Measure Handwashing Behavior? Use of Acceleration Sensors Embedded in Soap to Assess Reactivity to Structured Observation." *American Journal of Tropical Medicine and Hygiene* 83 (5): 1070–76.

Ram, P. K., I. Jahid, A. K. Halder, B. Nygren, M. S. Islam, S. P. Granger, J. W. Molyneaux, and S. P. Luby. 2011. "Variability in Hand Contamination Based on Serial Measurements: Implications for Assessment of Hand-Cleansing Behavior and Disease Risk." *The American Journal of Tropical Medicine and Hygiene* 84 (4): 510–16.

Ribot, J. C., and N. L. Peluso. 2003. "A Theory of Access." *Rural Sociology* 68 (2): 153–81.

Robiarto, A., E. Sofyan, D. Setiawan, A. Malina, and E. Rand. 2014. "Scaling Up Indonesia's Rural Sanitation Mobile Monitoring System Nationally." Water and Sanitation Program: Learning Note. World Bank, Washington, DC.

Sagerman, D., F. Nizame, J. Yu, S. P. Luby, and P. Ram. 2011. "Impact of Complexity of Instructions on Handwashing Adherence in a Low Income Setting." Presented at the American Society of Tropical Medical and Hygiene Conference Annual Meeting, December 4-8.

Schwemlein, S., R. Cronk, and J. Bartram. 2016. "Indicators for Monitoring Water, Sanitation, and Hygiene: A Systematic Review of Indicator Selection Methods." *International Journal of Environmental Research and Public Health* 13 (3): 333.

Sinha, A., C. L. Nagel, E. Thomas, W. P. Schmidt, B. Torondel, S. Boisson, and T. F. Clasen. 2016. "Assessing Latrine Use in Rural India: A Cross-Sectional Study Comparing Reported Use and Passive Latrine Use Monitors." *American Journal of Tropical Medicine and Hygiene* 95 (3): 720–27.

Thomas, E. A., and K. Mattson. 2013. "Instrumented Monitoring with Traditional Public Health Evaluation Methods: An Application to a Water, Sanitation and Hygiene Program in Jakarta, Indonesia." Mercy Corps, Portland, OR.

Webb, A. L., A. D. Stein, U. Ramakrishnan, V. S. Hertzberg, M. Urizar, and R. Martorell. 2006. "A Simple Index to Measure Hygiene Behaviours." *International Journal of Epidemiology* 35 (6): 1469–77.

WHO/UNICEF (World Health Organization/United Nations Children's Fund Joint Monitoring Programme for Water and Sanitation). 2015. *JMP Green Paper: Global Monitoring of Water, Sanitation and Hygiene Post-2015.* Geneva: WHO.

———. 2017. *Progress on Drinking Water, Sanitation, and Hygiene: 2017 Update and SDG Baselines.* Geneva: WHO.

CHAPTER 4

Behavioral Monitoring

Katie Fankhauser

Introduction

Measurement of the adoption and proper use of water and sanitation services is important to accurately report on Sustainable Development Goal 6 indicators. These measurements must extend beyond coverage of infrastructure to quantify actual usage of water and sanitation services. Studies have found that without high and consistent adherence by users programs for water treatment (Brown and Clasen 2012), sanitation (Clasen et al. 2014), and handwashing (Curtis, Danquah, and Aunger 2009) have little health benefit.

The behavioral measurement tools used by implementers are often chosen on the basis of cultural context, technical capacity, and resource availability (Biran et al. 2008; Ram et al. 2010). However, some monitoring standards have been established and will be outlined in this chapter. Many methods present challenges, including subjectivity (Biran et al. 2008; Ram 2013), reactivity (Ram et al. 2010), repeatability, cost, and skill. To address these issues, this chapter highlights newer technology-based monitoring methods that may provide a more objective indicator for measurement of water supply, sanitation, and hygiene (WASH) usage (see chapters 5 and 6 for further description of these methods).

Sector Guidance in Measuring WASH Usage

Many WASH evaluations are conducted through the use of survey-based self-reporting and proxy indicators. Survey-based tools are the most common and widely accepted method for data collection. The most comprehensive surveys follow principles of survey design and administration such as the use of non-leading questions, ensuring questions are contextually and culturally appropriate, and including observable measurements to reduce respondent bias. Furthermore, refining questions to specific, near-time periods can help reduce overestimation (Sinha et al. 2016), and asking covert questions that avoid asking directly about the behavior of interest can help mitigate over-reporting (Contzen, De Pasquale, and Mosler 2015). Because reactivity to repeated questioning can occur, researchers can also limit the number and frequency of surveys conducted on one individual, preferring larger sample sizes to smaller sample sizes with recurrent visits (Zwane et al. 2011).

Additional guidance in a specific sector has been found to further increase the quality of survey design. For example, in household water treatment programs, the World Health Organization published the *Toolkit for Monitoring and Evaluating Household Water Treatment and Safe Storage Programmes* (WHO and UNICEF 2012). The *Toolkit* outlines specific guidance on important survey questions as well as the wording of questions. The U.S. Agency for International Development has a manual for its Hygiene Improvement Project that favors objective spot checks and tests (USAID 2010).

Finally, another common method in measuring usage is through the use of direct, or structured, observation, in which an objective outsider records targeted activities within a household for a certain amount of time. This often serves as the gold standard to which other methods are compared.

Common Methods to Monitor WASH Usage

Self-Reports

Self-reported monitoring relies on direct responses from individuals whose behavior is of interest. Most commonly, it requires the use of an oral questionnaire conducted by an enumerator in the target setting, but respondents can also be asked to record their daily activities in a diary (Contzen, De Pasquale, and Mosler 2015) or on a calendar, or to be part of a focus group. Questions that are open-ended, close-ended, or scaled attempt to measure a variety of outcomes: baseline behavior and behavior change, WASH knowledge, awareness of an intervention, and determinants of behavior that include access, ability, and motivation (Ram 2013).

Self-reports are the easiest and most common monitoring schemes. The ability to create one centralized survey that can reach large numbers of people at relatively low cost makes it an efficient method. It also offers evaluators a degree of quality control if the survey is delivered systematically over the program region.

However, as described elsewhere in this report (see chapter 1), self-reports are often limited by over-reporting and bias. Survey questionnaires can be used to evaluate exposure to an intervention by assessing the level of awareness and knowledge of the population to the target behavior and to elucidate factors that may encourage or hinder WASH behaviors (Ram 2013). As such they can be useful to inform programmatic planning and adjustments, but they should not be relied upon to give objective measures of behavior change or intervention performance.

Proxy Indicators

Proxy indicators, also called rapid observation or spot checks, are inclusive of many techniques. By definition they do not aim to observe actual actions but instead measure outcomes that are known to be associated with the target usage behavior. For example, with latrines this means looking for a well-worn path, wet floor, odor, and the presence of flies, feces, and anal-cleansing materials in and around the latrine (Clasen et al. 2012). Observation of enablers of and barriers to usage of a WASH system, such as presence of soap or ability to quickly retrieve it, proximity of a designated washing area to the toilet and kitchen, and water availability, serve as proxy indicators for handwashing. Presence of water in the filter, correct demonstrations of use and maintenance, and water quality tests, including presence of chlorine, are indicators commonly used to measure household water treatment practices (USAID 2010; Rosa et al. 2014b; Barstow et al. 2016).

Spot checks provide a less intrusive alternative to direct observation and induce less reactivity from subjects (Ruel and Arimond 2002). Spot checks can also be easily incorporated into household surveys, including monitoring programs that often have both types of metrics. For example, large Demographic and Health Surveys, such as the multi-indicator cluster survey of the United Nations Children's Fund, monitor handwashing with soap by asking the enumerator to confirm the presence of soap and water at the handwashing station in addition to asking about usual hygiene practice (Ram 2013).

Considering the association of several indicators together to the target outcome could elucidate the magnitude and direction of the impact of an intervention. Creating composite indexes, which are less susceptible to inter-household variability and reactivity, may improve the accuracy of proxies to predict complex hygiene behaviors that involve multiple actions (Webb et al. 2006). Additionally, indexes can evaluate the reach of the intervention when the index includes select variables that are targeted by the intervention (Ruel and Arimond 2002).

Direct/Structured Observations

Structured observations have historically been a highly regarded monitoring method. Structured observations involve placing an observer near the activity of interest—for example, within a household, at a school, or outside a latrine—for a specified period of time (Halder et al. 2013). The observer records the behavior of interest and notes individuals' responses, such as drinking of filtered water or handwashing after defecation. It is important to schedule observations around critical times, when there is more opportunity to perform the desired action and most householders are at home, so that the behavior and individuals of interest are studied (Biran et al. 2008; Halder et al. 2013). Observations can be simply binary (Biran et al. 2008)—yes/no washed hands after fecal contact—or open-ended, allowing the observer to capture all possible detail about the event, such as type of soap used to wash hands (Ram 2013).

Structured observations, often incorporated as part of survey activities, can provide a fine grain of detail about habits, sequence of events, behavior during critical times, and how behavior differs among individuals and visitors in a household. Because data are collected on individuals, behavior can be analyzed across gender, age, and household role. Additionally, information about behavior around critical events, such as washing hands before food preparation and after defecation, is obtained. Finally, consistency in behavior can be measured through direct observation, determining whether an individual always uses a latrine to defecate, washes her hands afterward, or drinks treated water exclusively while the observer is present (Ram 2013; Rosa et al. 2014a).

Despite being what some consider the gold standard in WASH monitoring and evaluation, structured observation still has substantial limitations. First, implementation is resource intensive, requiring time, labor, and funds. Quality enumerators and comprehensive training are required to limit bias due to respondent reactivity and observer differences. This is especially important when the measurement is fairly subjective—inclusive of self-reported behaviors and proxy indicators, but also those dependent on observer interpretation—because this has been shown to bias effect estimates (Wood et al. 2008). Second, the length of time the observer is in the household may be inconvenient for study participants and may change their routine (Halder et al. 2013). Third, similar to survey reactivity, the act of repeated observation has been shown to augment the behavior of interest, known as the Hawthorne effect (Zwane et al. 2011). The presence of a human observer outside of a latrine modifies the usual behavior of households, significantly increasing the use of the latrine (Clasen et al. 2012). Similarly, one study showed soap use after crucial events is higher in the first 90 minutes of observation than in the following three and a half hours (Halder et al. 2013). Additionally, households with higher social status show more reactivity to the observer, meaning the exercise may capture information about the population differentially (Ram et al. 2010). Finally, direct observation has been shown to have low repeatability in individual monitoring and may be appropriate only to measure behavior at a population level or after repeated observations (Cousens et al. 1996), although the latter has the potential to produce a Hawthorne effect as well.

When performing structured observations, like all of the methods discussed so far, it is necessary to control for reactivity by not allowing subjects to know the type of data collected or for what purpose (Biran et al. 2008). Additional care is needed in assessing the duration of the observation. Longer periods are recommended because shorter observation periods can miss too many critical events and induce more reactivity from subjects (Halder et al. 2013).

Technology-Based Methods

A multitude of smartphone applications developed in the past few years allow enumerators to complete electronic surveys in the field and later upload the data remotely to a central database. Paperless data collection reduces transcription and delivery errors while collection and analysis time are reduced substantially. More rapid feedback gives programs the opportunity to adapt and improve their messaging so they have larger impact over the program period. Instrumentation, such as sensors monitoring water pump functionality and latrine or soap use, can provide increased data quality. Extensive review of data and sensor-based tools is provided in chapters 5 and 6.

Combined Methodologies

Given that all monitoring and evaluation methods have their own advantages and limitations, it is often beneficial to leverage more than one method to get a fuller picture of WASH behavior. Surveys, ethnographies, and direct observation give context to sensor readings. Sensors or spot checks may give a picture of household characteristics, but surveys and, ideally, structured observations are used to inform individual behavior, which further refines the algorithm or index for streamlined analysis during subsequent monitoring periods. When more than one monitoring method evaluates an intervention, it often suggests the validity of the others when correlation and mean differences between them are calculated. Overall, combined methodologies can provide a more comprehensive and instructive depiction of WASH usage.

An important function of sensors, reviewed in chapter 5, is their ability to validate the reliability of another method, while also suggesting improvements to standards of practice. For example, higher correlation between sensors and self-reports is seen when the questionnaire focuses on near-time behavior, in the previous 48 hours, suggesting how surveys should be administered in future studies (Sinha et al. 2016). The appropriateness of structured observation as the gold standard has been questioned through the use of sensors where Passive Latrine Use Monitors were used to show significant reactivity to the presence of an observer (Clasen et al. 2012). Similar findings were made with SmartSoap for handwashing behavior (Ram et al. 2010).

Conclusion

Of the various monitoring tools for measuring WASH usage outlined throughout this chapter, each has its own advantages, limitations, and proposed mitigation to ensure that reliability and validity are met. Reactivity may be the greatest challenge in evaluating water and sanitation proper use and adherence although new technology-based methods may provide some solutions. Overall, a combined methodology that incorporates a variety of methods will be helpful to limit or at least identify any potential biases.

References

Barstow, C. K., C. L. Nagel, T. F. Clasen, and E. A. Thomas. 2016. "Process Evaluation and Assessment of Use of a Large Scale Water Filter and Cookstove Program in Rwanda." *BMC Public Health* 16: 584.

Biran, A., T. Rabie, W. Schmidt, S. Juvekar, S. Hirve, and V. Curtis. 2008. "Comparing the Performance of Indicators Of Hand-Washing Practices in Rural Indian Households." *Tropical Medicine and International Health* 13 (2): 278–85.

Brown, J., and T. Clasen. 2012. "High Adherence Is Necessary to Realize Health Gains from Water Quality Interventions." *PLoS ONE* 7 (5): e36735.

Clasen, T., S. Boisson, P. Routray, B. Torondel, M. Bell, O. Cumming, J. Ensink, M. Freeman, M. Jenkins, M. Odagiri, S. Ray, A. Sinha, M. Suar, and W.-P. Schmidt. 2014. "Effectiveness of a Rural Sanitation Programme on Diarrhoea, Soil-Transmitted Helminth Infection, and Child Malnutrition in Odisha, India: A Cluster-Randomised Trial." *The Lancet Global Health* 2 (11): e645–53.

Clasen, T., D. Fabini, S. Boisson, J. Taneja, J. Song, E. Aichinger, A. Bui, S. Dadashi, W. P. Schmidt, Z. Burt, and K. L. Nelson. 2012. "Making Sanitation Count: Developing and Testing a Device for Assessing Latrine Use in Low-Income Settings." *Environmental Science and Technology* 46 (6): 3295–303.

Contzen, N., S. De Pasquale, and H. J. Mosler. 2015. "Over-Reporting in Handwashing Self-Reports: Potential Explanatory Factors and Alternative Measurements." *PLoS ONE* 10 (8): 1–22.

Cousens, S., B. Kanki, S. Toure, I. Diallo, and V. Curtis. 1996. "Reactivity and Repeatability of Hygiene Behaviour: Structured Observations from Burkina Faso." *Social Science and Medicine* 43 (9): 1299–308.

Curtis, V. A., L. O. Danquah, and R. V. Aunger. 2009. "Planned, Motivated and Habitual Hygiene Behaviour: An Eleven Country Review." *Health Education Research* 24 (4): 655–73.

Halder, A. K., J. W. Molyneaux, S. P. Luby, and P. K. Ram. 2013. "Impact of Duration of Structured Observations on Measurement of Handwashing Behavior at Critical Times." *BMC Public Health* 13: 705.

Ram, P. 2013. "Practical Guidance for Measuring Handwashing Behavior: 2013 Update." Water and Sanitation Working Paper, World Bank, Washington, DC.

Ram, P. K., A. K. Halder, S. P. Granger, T. Jones, P. Hall, D. Hitchcock, R. Wright, B. Nygren, M. S. Islam, J. W. Molyneaux, and S. P. Luby. 2010. "Is Structured Observation a Valid Technique to Measure Handwashing Behavior? Use of Acceleration Sensors Embedded in Soap to Assess Reactivity to Structured Observation." *American Journal of Tropical Medicine and Hygiene* 83 (5): 1070–76.

Rosa, G., M. L. Huaylinos, A. Gil, C. Lanata, and T. Clasen. 2014a. "Assessing the Consistency and Microbiological Effectiveness of Household Water Treatment Practices by Urban and Rural Populations Claiming to Treat their Water at Home: A Case Study in Peru." *PLoS ONE* 9 (12): 1–19.

Rosa, G., F. Majorin, S. Boisson, C. Barstow, M. Johnson, M. Kirby, F. Ngabo, E. Thomas, and T. Clasen. 2014b. "Assessing the Impact of Water Filters and Improved Cook Stoves on Drinking Water Quality and Household Air Pollution: A Randomised Controlled Trial in Rwanda." *PLoS ONE* 9 (3): 1–9.

Ruel, M. T., and M. Arimond. 2002. "Spot-Check Observations for Assessing Hygiene Practices: Review of Experience and Implications for Programs." *Journal of Health, Population and Nutrition* 20 (1): 65–76.

Sinha, A., C. L. Nagel, E. Thomas, W. P. Schmidt, B. Torondel, S. Boisson, and T. F. Clasen. 2016. "Assessing Latrine Use in Rural India: A Cross-Sectional Study Comparing

Reported Use and Passive Latrine Use Monitors." *American Journal of Tropical Medicine and Hygiene* 95 (3): 720–27.

USAID (U.S. Agency for International Development). 2010. "Access and Behavioral Outcome Indicators for Water, Sanitation, and Hygiene." Hygiene Improvement Project, USAID, Washington, DC.

Webb, A. L., A. D. Stein, U. Ramakrishnan, V. S. Hertzberg, M. Urizar, and R. Martorell. 2006. "A Simple Index to Measure Hygiene Behaviours." *International Journal of Epidemiology* 35 (6): 1469–77.

WHO (World Health Organization) and UNICEF (United Nations Children's Fund). 2012. *A Toolkit for Monitoring and Evaluating Household Water Treatment and Safe Storage Programmes.* Geneva: WHO.

Wood, L., M. Egger, L. L. Gluud, K. F. Schulz, P. Jüni, D. G. Altman, C. Gluud, R. M. Martin, A. J. G. Wood, and J. A. C. Sterne. 2008. "Empirical Evidence of Bias in Treatment Effect Estimates in Controlled Trials with Different Interventions and Outcomes: Meta-Epidemiological Study." *British Medical Journal* 336 (7644): 601–05.

Zwane, A. P., J. Zinman, E. V. Dusen, W. Pariente, C. Null, E. Miguel, M. Kremer, D. S. Karlan, R. Hornbeck, X. Giné, E. Duflo, F. Devoto, B. Crepon, and A. Banerjee. 2011. "Being Surveyed Can Change Later Behavior and Related Parameter Estimates." *Proceedings of the National Academy of Sciences* 108 (5): 1821–26.

CHAPTER 5

Sensing WASH—In Situ and Remote Sensing Technologies

Evan Thomas

Introduction

The resilience of water and sanitation services is dependent upon credible and continuous indicators of reliability, leveraged by funding agencies to incentivize performance among service providers. In many countries, these service providers are utilities providing access to clean water and safe sanitation. However, in emerging economies, there often remains a significant gap between the intent of service providers and the impacts delivered over time.

Remote monitoring, via satellite assets and in situ sensors, may offer some contribution to addressing some of the challenges of information asymmetry and data gaps in developing communities including unreliable survey data and relying on spot checks to assess performance. Data can be used to understand programmatic, social, economic, and seasonal changes that may influence the quality of a program. Additionally, behavioral patterns of the user can be studied to better understand how and when the water and sanitation technologies are being used. In this chapter we review the use of remote sensing and local sensors for water, sanitation, and hygiene (WASH) monitoring.

The term remote sensing usually describes the collection of data by satellites. In most cases, the "remote" refers to spectral imagery collected by cameras and other spectral instruments across a broad range of wavelengths. In the case of Earth observation, satellites take spectral data reflecting from the atmosphere and the Earth's surface. Interpretation of this data (often represented as imagery) requires an understanding of spectral data and physical properties of the Earth and atmosphere. It also often requires calibration against data collected on the Earth's surface or in the atmosphere directly—data from sensors that are in situ, rather than remote.

In situ instrumentation technologies vary from flow meters and water quality sensors to motion detectors installed in latrines. These sensor technologies can be used operationally or within a statistical sampling frame. Data can be logged locally for manual retrieval or transmitted over short range to nearby enumerators, or to remote operators and researchers over Wi-Fi, cellular, satellite, and other wireless networks. Some instrumentation is in common use, whereas other technologies are emerging. However, given the remote and power-constrained environments and the high degree of variability between fixed infrastructure including age, materials, quality, servicing, and functionality, any electronic sensor–based solution often either is custom engineering or compensates for these complexities through analytics. For example, a conventional flow meter designed for a rural borehole water distribution scheme would have to address pipe diameter, material, pressure, depth, thread type, and other characteristics that require custom engineering and plumbing. Instead, a nonintrusive ultrasonic flow meter may be more easily adapted for a variety of water schemes.

Satellite Remote Sensing

Remote sensing capabilities and techniques are well suited for monitoring regional-scale precipitation, water budgets, soil moisture, and some measures of water quality. A recent World Bank report summarized the water resource management applications of remote sensing:

> Remote sensing plays an increasingly important role in providing the information needed to confront key water challenges. In poorly gauged basins, at time intervals of several days, real-time satellite estimates of precipitation and derived streamflow forecasts can help managers to allocate water among users and to operate reservoirs more efficiently. In large rivers, data on river and lake surface elevation can be used to estimate flow in the upper parts of the basin and to predict flow downstream. Soil moisture observations may give insight into how much irrigation is needed, as well as help to forecast and monitor drought conditions. Water managers in snow-dominated areas can use estimates of snow cover and snow water equivalent to assess how much water is in storage and determine what watersheds it is stored in. Remote sensing also enables the monitoring of many parameters of surface water quality to assess the repercussions of river basin management policies, land use practices, and nonpoint source pollution as well as the likelihood of algal blooms and other threats to the quality of water supply systems. (Garcia et al. 2016)

A variety of satellite data products have been leveraged to aid water and sanitation programs. Key examples include the following:

- The Landsat program of the National Aeronautics and Space Administration (NASA) and the U.S. Geological Survey was launched in 1972 and was the first Earth observation satellite designed for public use. Landsat 8, launched in 2013, has two primary instruments, the Operational Land Imager (visible, near infrared [IR] and shortwave IR) and the Thermal Infrared Sensor (TIRS). Landsat 8 covers every point on Earth every 16 days, and has a resolution of 15–100 meters. TIRS was added to the Landsat 8 mission "when it became clear that state water resource managers rely on the highly accurate measurements of Earth's thermal energy obtained by LDCM's [Landsat Data Continuity

Mission] predecessors, Landsat 5 and Landsat 7, to track how land and water are being used."[1]

In particular, Landsat 8 data allows the calculation of the Normalized Differential Vegetation Index (NDVI). Landsat 8 NDVI allows an estimation of land surface emissivity (Sobrino, Jiménez-Muñoz, and Paolini 2004) and land cover classification (Weng, Lu, and Schubring 2004) as well as surface temperature. Remote sensing experts can use these measures for planning-level estimation of watershed health across a broad region. Additionally, land use classification can identify rural versus urban built environment and population density.

- SERVIR, a cooperative initiative of NASA and the U.S. Agency for International Development (USAID), "works in partnership with leading regional organizations world-wide to help developing countries use information provided by Earth observing satellites and geospatial technologies for managing climate risks and land use."[2] With three regional offices, SERVIR has been able to partner with remote sensing experts and national decision-making bodies. Among other activities, SERVIR focuses on monitoring bodies of water to observe effects from "human activities, climate change, and other environmental phenomena." SERVIR takes advantage of Landsat, ASTER, MODIS (Moderate Resolution Imaging Spectroradiometer), and other satellite assets to monitor water quality and changes. Specifically, SERVIR is developing rainfall and runoff models to study the availably and quality of surface water over the next several decades.

- Using Tropic Rainfall Measuring Mission data, the Nile Basin Initiative in partnership with NASA provides flood forecasts and water balance estimates for the Eastern Nile basin. Similarly, the Land Surface Hydrology Group at Princeton University developed the Africa Drought Monitor and provides maps of rainfall, temperature, and other hydrologic variables (Garcia et al. 2016).

- The USAID Famine Early Warning System Network (FEWS NET) monitors rainfall and crop production with satellite assets and combines these data with socioeconomic insights to identify population groups that may be vulnerable to food insecurity.[3]

- NASA's Terra satellite includes two instruments that have been leveraged for watershed monitoring. MODIS and the Multiangle Imaging Spectroradiometer satellite assets can be used to determine aerosol optical depth, land surface temperature, enhanced vegetation index, and middle IR reflectance. Some of these data can be used to assess water quality parameters including chlorophyll, cyanobacterial pigments, colored dissolved organic matter, and suspended matter on a large water body scale (Garcia et al. 2016).

- In Nigeria, the World Bank recently used geographic information system mapping techniques to compare household survey data against MODIS land use estimates to generate spatial distribution estimates of water and sanitation indicators, including water and sanitation service access (World Bank 2017).

- The Inter-American Development Bank (IDB) developed the Hydro-BID platform to assist countries in Latin America and the Caribbean with water management through the mapping and tracking of over 230,000 water catchment areas. The Hydro-BID platform is leveraged by government agencies and water utilities for regional water management and infrastructure planning.[4]

Unmanned Aerial Vehicles

Increasingly, researchers are using unmanned aerial vehicles (UAVs, or drones) to map watersheds. Structure from motion three-dimensional point clouds can be derived from digital images collected by UAVs, similar to the type of data produced by Light Detection and Ranging (LiDAR) technology (Harwin and Lucieer 2012). The technological development of UAVs and their ability to derive high-resolution three-dimensional information at a much lower operational and up-front cost than manned airborne platforms and satellite imaging has made UAV image acquisition appealing in several applications. Research applications using UAVs for environmental monitoring, management, and evaluation have been increasingly explored in the past 10 years. The use of UAVs for data collection in natural resource (Horcher and Visser 2004; Laliberte et al. 2010), biomass (Dufour et al. 2013), forest (Koh and Wich 2012; Fritz, Kattenborn, and Koch 2013; Zarco-Tejada et al. 2014), and vegetation (Dandois and Ellis 2013; Salami, Barrado, and Pastor 2014) monitoring has been found to have significant impacts on the temporal and spatial resolution of data at a more cost-effective price than traditional monitoring practices.

Water Quality Sensors

Several water quality sensors are commonly used for both in situ continuous monitoring and sample-based testing. Off-the-shelf sensors are readily available to measure pH, dissolved oxygen, conductivity (often used to measure salinity), turbidity, temperature, chlorine, and various dissolved ions including fluoride, ammonia, silver, nitrates and nitrites (often byproducts of fertilizers), and total organic carbon. A complete review of these sensors and their applications is outside the scope of this report.

Instead, several more recent sensor applications, directly relevant to Sustainable Development Goal (SDG) targets 6.1 and 6.2 monitoring, are highlighted.

Microbial Sensors

- A class of optical fluorimeters offers a potential for real-time in situ fecal contamination detection. These sensors detect tryptophan-like fluorescence (TLF) associated with the presence of microbial contamination. In recent years, several laboratory-grade products have been validated in the field as predictive of *Escherichia coli* (*E. coli*) (Baker et al. 2015; Sorensen et al. 2015). However, these instruments require frequent cleaning, are not intended for long-term autonomous operation, and cost $7,500 or more.

These state-of-the-art fluorimeter solutions are not designed for long-term in situ use, primarily because of biofouling and baseline drift that attenuate and ambiguate the signal (Coble et al. 2014). At present, there are no viable in situ electronic sensors for monitoring microbial contamination of drinking water. The closest products suitable for this application are spectroscopy-based sensors for TLF from *E. coli*. The United Nations Children's Fund has recently published a Target Product Profile detailing a market need for improved sensor systems for microbial contamination in drinking water (UNICEF 2014).

Chemical Sensors

- Fluoride monitoring is also a priority chemical constituent in some countries. There are several commercially available sensor products for fluoride monitoring including the Hach sensION+ Fluoride Ion Electrode and various in-line sensors for larger-scale water distribution systems, such as the Rosemount Fluoride Monitoring System (Emerson Automated Solutions 2017), and the ATI Fluoride Monitor.[5]
- In Bangladesh, where arsenic contamination is a priority contaminant affecting health, a collaborative of researchers and practitioners is developing and testing biosensors that can be rapidly deployed to indicate arsenic contamination in drinking water.[6]
- Similarly, there are several off-the-shelf sensor-based technologies for monitoring arsenic contamination. These include the Palintest Digital Arsenic Test Kit[7] and the IPI Digital Arsenic Detector.[8] However, there remains a need for additional technology development in this area, as highlighted by the recent U.S. Environmental Protection Agency Arsenic Sensor Prize Competition (McAllister 2016).

Multi-Parameter Sensors

- Akvo Caddisfly builds on the smartphone-based application Akvo Flow, a survey-based application similar to smartphone and dashboard programs described in chapter 6.[9] Currently Akvo Caddisfly can measure several water quality parameters. Fluoride is measured by collecting water in a test chamber, adding a reagent to the sample, and taking a photo to analyze the concentration according to the color generated by the sample and reagent mixture. Salinity is measured with an electrical conductivity sensor attached directly to the phone via a USB cable. Additionally, any color-based test strip can be analyzed by Akvo Caddisfly automatically corresponding the test strip color to the color calibration card, thereby taking out any subjectivity on the part of the user.

Water Service Delivery and Use

In municipal water supplies in many cities, water flow meters are commonly used to measure service delivery and enable billing. These meters vary in functionality and form, from manually read mechanical meters to remotely reporting sensors. A challenge facing water service providers and customers is "non-revenue water" (NRW)—water that is produced but not billed for. In developing countries, NRW is estimated at more than $40 billion per year, losing enough water to serve 200 million people—45 billion liters—and a further 30 billion liters lost to poor metering or billing processes. This negative feedback loop diminishes the capacity of utilities to deliver reliable, safe water, and the willingness of customers to pay for this service.

- Improved water meters and processes can reduce this NRW gap, and improve the quality and faith in water service delivery. In India, NextDrop Technologies has combined remotely reporting water meters with periodic water quality tests to reduce water consumption, leaks, and service outages.[10]

- Also in India, the social enterprise Piramal Sarvajal developed a reverse osmosis water treatment "ATM" (automated teller machine) that continuously monitors and remotely reports on system functionality and water quality.[11]

- In Sub-Saharan Africa, about one million hand pumps supply water to over 200 million rural water users across the continent, yet as many as one-third of all hand pumps are thought not to be working at any given time, with 30–70 percent broken within two years. In 2013, Oxford University conducted trials on 66 mobile-enabled "smart hand pumps." The study demonstrated that hand pumps with cellular network–enabled sensors that were repaired in the trial saw a decrease in pump downtime from an average of 27 days to 2.6 days. Participating communities also increased by over threefold their willingness to pay for pump services (Koehler, Thomson, and Hope 2015).

- Building on this work, in 2014, Portland State University and Living Water International installed 181 cellular-enabled water pump use sensors in three provinces of Rwanda (photo 5.1 shows these sensors in use in Kenya). The nominal maintenance model was compared against a "best practice" circuit rider model, wherein dedicated staff and supplies were assigned to pump groups, and an "ambulance" service model wherein sensor data triggered

Photo 5.1 SweetSense Inc. Water Pump Sensors Installed in Western Kenya

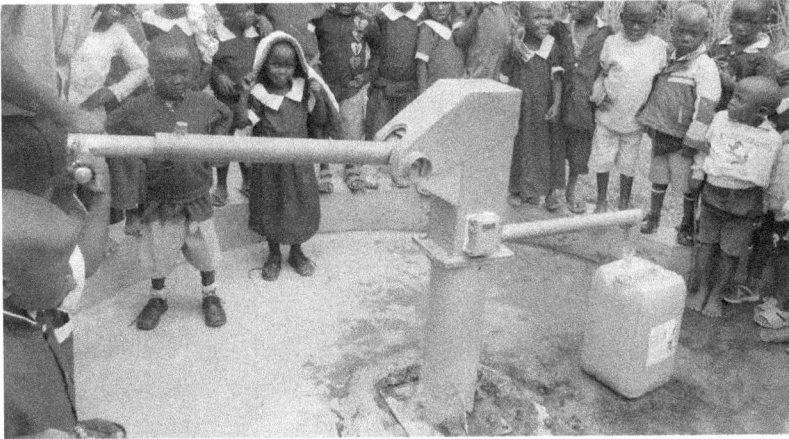

a service dispatch. In only the ambulance model were the sensor data available to the implementer and used to dispatch technicians. In the baseline, 56 percent of the implementer's pumps were functional, with a mean reported non-functionality of approximately 214 days. In the study period, the nominal maintenance group had a median time to successful repair of approximately 152 days, with a mean per-pump functionality of about 68 percent. In the circuit rider group, the median time to successful repair was nearly 57 days, with a per-pump functionality mean of nearly 73 percent. In the ambulance service group the successful repair interval was nearly 21 days with a functionality mean of nearly 91 percent (Nagel et al. 2015).

- Smart metering, an approach first matured in the power industry, allows a water utility to obtain meter readings on demand without requiring manual meter readers. A recent IDB report summarized the opportunities and limitations of smart water meters (Arniella 2016). Smart meters can benefit the water utility, the environment, and the utility's customers by
  - Lowering the cost of meter reading by eliminating manual meter reading;
  - Enhancing employee safety by reducing the number of personnel on the road;
  - Reducing billing errors and disputes;
  - Monitoring the water system in a timely manner;
  - Enabling flexible reading schedules, reducing delays in billing of commercial accounts;
  - Providing useful data for balancing customer demand;
  - Enabling possible dynamic pricing (raising or lowering the cost of water according to demand, promotions, and customer incentives);
  - Benefitting the environment by reducing pollution from vehicles driven by meter readers;

- Assessing NRW in real time or short intervals;
- Facilitating the data to establish the night water consumption patterns, analyzing the minimum night flows, and offering a more detailed feedback on water use patterns;
- Enabling customers to adjust their habits to lower water bills;
- Providing real-time billing information, reducing estimated readings and re-billing costs;
- Reducing customer complaint calls and increasing customer satisfaction;
- Improving the monitoring of potential meter tampering and water theft; and
- Detecting water line leaks sooner, so they can be repaired faster.

Although smart meters have many benefits, they also present challenges to water utilities, customers, and the environment. They require
- Front-end capital investment;
- Long-term financial commitment to the new metering technology and related software;
- Ensuring the security of metering data and preventing cyberattacks;
- Transitioning to new technology and processes with proper training;
- Managing public reaction and customer acceptance of the new meters;
- Managing and storing vast quantities of metering data; and
- Disposing of the old meters.

- Similarly, MoMo (mobile monitor) is a mobile device that can be integrated with physical sensors to track infrastructure and improve accountability in the developing world.[12] The MoMo platform is open source, and the technology incorporates a modular design so that it can be used for a variety of applications. Although the first applications of MoMo have focused on measuring flow rates on rural hand pumps, the website indicates that MoMo sensor boards can support up to 100 logical sensors related to pulse counting, voltage, current, pressure readings, or serial communication. Given the focus on rural applications in remote areas, the MoMo device is optimized for low-power use to preserve battery life. Data are recorded from sensors according to a user-specified sample rate, and the board controller aggregates the data for transmission over cellular networks. Data are then stored on servers for processing, analysis, and communication of information through online portals or automated Short Message Service (SMS) messages. An early application of the MoMo device was used to monitor the flow rate of water in rural hand pumps using SMS messages to transmit data to their servers. However, inadequate network coverage in the area where the sensors were installed resulted in a high proportion of the messages being lost (Pearce, Dickinson, and Welle 2015).

- In two recently funded USAID programs in Ethiopia (USAID 2016) and Kenya (USAID 2015), sensors connected to the satellite network are being installed on remote electrically powered boreholes to monitor functionality and water service delivery, each to thousands of customers. These measures will be entered into decision aids that may dispatch technicians, supplies, or other response.

Household Water Treatment Use

- Several products are available commercially to monitor residual chlorine, an indication of water treatment practices and water safety. These include pocket colorimeters from Hach,[13] Analyticon,[14] DKK-TOA,[15] Omega,[16] and other vendors.

- The use of household water filters has also been measured in some studies. In Rwanda, a cluster randomized controlled trial was conducted among 170 households (70 blinded to the presence of the sensor, 100 open) testing whether awareness of an electronic monitor would result in a difference in weekly use of household water over a four-week surveillance period. A 63 percent increase in the number of uses of the water filter per week between the groups was observed in week 1, an average of 4.4 times in the open group and 2.83 times in the blind group, declining in week 4 to an insignificant 55 percent difference of 2.82 uses in the open, and 1.93 in the blind. Use of the water filters decreased in both groups over four-week installation periods. This study suggests behavioral monitoring should attempt to account for reactivity to awareness of electronic monitors that persists for weeks or more (Thomas et al. 2016).

Sanitation Use

In several sections of this report, a motion detector–based sensor platform for estimating latrine use is described (see chapters 3 and 4). In several studies, the technology used is the Passive Latrine Use Monitor (PLUM) first developed at the University of California at Berkeley (Clasen et al. 2012). The sensor uses a simple passive IR motion detector to identify warm-bodied movement in a latrine stall. This binary movement data is recorded at three-second intervals, and either logged locally on the sensor device or transmitted by cellular or satellite data networks for online processing. Structured observation validated algorithms process this movement data into discrete use estimates. These estimates have been shown to be more reliable at individual households than in community latrines where lines may form. In some cases, the sensors include radio frequency identification readers to enable latrine-servicing requests, as demonstrated with Sanergy Inc., in Nairobi, Kenya.

In one recent study in Bangladesh, these sensors demonstrated a significant over-reporting of latrine use. Across 1,207 households randomly selected from 52 village committees in Bangladesh, the mean four-day self-reported number of latrine uses was 32.8, whereas sensor analysis suggested 21.7 uses on average, indicating more than 50 percent exaggeration of latrine use. At the low end of the regression model, the intercept suggests that many households report using latrines when in fact no use is detected (Delea et al. 2017). Similarly, in a recent cross-sectional study among 292 households in 25 villages in India, these sensors were installed for two weeks and compared to household responded surveys. The mean reported daily use was nearly twice that of the sensor-recorded use with moderate agreement between daily reported use over the past 48 hours (Sinha et al. 2016).

Handwashing Monitoring

Sensors can also provide an objective and nonobtrusive characterization of handwashing behavior.

- SmartSoap, developed by Unilever, is an ordinary looking bar of soap with an embedded accelerometer that measures motion on three axes, allowing the detection of use. On its own, SmartSoap can provide an accurate count of the number of times the soap bar is used each day. By combining SmartSoap data with data from a motion sensor placed on the vessel holding water for anal cleansing, researchers were able to detect handwashing events after defecation. Although overall soap use increased, they found that there was no increase in the number of soap uses following defecation (Ram 2010).

- Similarly, Mercy Corps used motion detector–based latrine sensors combined with water flow sensors to monitor the prevalence of handwashing after latrine use. They found that water use after latrine use was very low (less than 10 percent) in all but one district, which registered almost 40 percent use of water after latrine use. They also found that self-reported use of the latrine and handwashing after using the latrine was much greater (up to 4 times and 25 times, respectively) than the latrine use and handwashing after latrine use detected by the sensors (Thomas and Mattson 2013).

Notes

1. Taken from the NASA website. For more information, visit https://landsat.gsfc.nasa.gov/thermal-infrared-sensor-tirs/.
2. Taken from the SERVIR Global website. For more information, visit https://www.servirglobal.net.
3. More information is available from the FEWS NET website, http://www.fews.net/content/using-crowdsourcing-map-displacement-south-sudan.
4. More information on the Hydro-BID simulation tool is available on the Hydrobid website, http://hydrobidlac.org.
5. More information on the ATI Flouride Monitor is available on the Analytical Technology, Inc. website, https://www.analyticaltechnology.com/analyticaltechnology/gas-water-monitors/product.aspx?ProductID=1052.
6. For more information, see the partnership's website, www.arsenicbiosensor.org.

7. More information about the kit is available on Palintest's website, http://www .palintest.com/en/products/digital-arsenic-test-kit.

8. For more information on the IPI's arsenic monitoring equipment, see the IPI Singapore website, https://www.ipi-singapore.org/tags/arsenic-monitoring-analysis-sensor -measurement-equipment.

9. Information on Akvo Caddisfly comes from the Akvo Foundation website, http:// akvo.org/akvo-caddisfly/.

10. For more information on NextDrop Technologies and the NextDrop Water Marketplace, see NextDrop's website, nextdrop.co.

11. More information about Piramal Sarvajal's water solutions is available on its website, http://www.sarvajal.com.

12. More information about the MoMo platform and its applications is available on MoMo's website, http://momo.welldone.org/about/.

13. For more information about the Hach colorimeter, see the company's website, https:// www.hach.com/colorimeters/dr900-colorimeter/family?productCategoryId =35547203827.

14. More information about the Analyticon Residual Chlorine Meter is available on the company's website, http://www.analyticon.com/products/portable-handheld-meters /Residual-Chlorine-Meter-Low-range-0-2ppm.php.

15. For more information about DKK-TOA, see the company's website, http://www .dkktoa.com.co/news/2011/4/30/model-rc-31p-hand-held-residual-chlorine-meter .html.

16. For more information, see Omega's website, http://www.omega.com/pptst/CLH1740 .html.

References

Arniella, E. F. 2016. *Evaluation of Smart Water Infrastructure Technologies (SWIT)*. Washington, DC: Inter-American Development Bank.

Baker, A., S. A. Cumberland, C. Bradley, C. Buckley, and J. Bridgeman. 2015. "To What Extent Can Portable Fluorescence Spectroscopy Be Used in the Real-Time Assessment of Microbial Water Quality?" *Science of the Total Environment* 532 (November): 14–19.

Clasen, T., D. Fabini, S. Boisson, J. Taneja, J. Song, E. Aichinger, A. Bui, S. Dadashi, W. P. Schmidt, Z. Burt, and K. L. Nelson. 2012. "Making Sanitation Count: Developing and Testing a Device for Assessing Latrine Use in Low-Income Settings." *Environmental Science & Technology* 46 (6): 3295–303.

Coble, P. G., J. Lead, A. Baker, D. M. Reynolds, and R. G. M. Spencer. 2014. *Aquatic Organic Matter Fluorescence*. New York, NY: Cambridge University Press.

Dandois, J. P., and E. C. Ellis. 2013. "High Spatial Resolution Three-Dimensional Mapping of Vegetation Spectral Dynamics Using Computer Vision." *Remote Sensing of Environment* 136 (September): 259–76.

Delea, M. C. Nagel, E. Thomas, A. Halder, N. Amin, A. Shoab, M. Freeman, L. Unicomb, and T. Clasen. 2017. "Comparison of Respondent-Reported and Sensor-Recorded Latrine Utilization Measures in Rural Bangladesh: A Cross-Sectional Study." *Transactions of the Royal Society of Tropical Medicine and Hygiene*. https://doi .org/10.1093/trstmh/trx058.

Dufour, S., I. Bernez, J. Betbeder, S. Corgne, L. Hubert-Moy, J. Nabucet, S. Rapinel, J. Sawtschuk, and C. Trollè. 2013. "Monitoring Restored Riparian Vegetation: How Can Recent Developments in Remote Sensing Sciences Help?" *Knowledge and Management of Aquatic Ecosystems* 410 (10): 1–15.

Emerson Automated Solutions. 2017. "Floride Monitoring System." Data Product Sheet, Emerson Automated Solutions, Shakopee, MN, June.

Fritz, A., T. Kattenborn, and B. Koch. 2013. "UAV-Based Photogrammetric Point Clouds— Tree Stem Mapping in Open Stands in Comparison to Terrestrial Laser Scanner Point Clouds." *International Archives of the Photogrammetry, Remote Sensing and Spatial Information Sciences* XL-1/W2: 141–46.

Garcia, L. E., D. J. Rodríguez, M. Wijnen, and I. Pakulski. 2016. *Earth Observation for Water Resources Management.* Washington, DC: World Bank Group.

Harwin, S., and A. Lucieer. 2012. "Assessing the Accuracy of Georeferenced Point Clouds Produced via Multi-View Stereopsis from Unmanned Aerial Vehicle (UAV) Imagery." *Remote Sensing* 4 (6): 1573–99.

Horcher, A., and R. J. M. Visser. 2004. "Unmanned Aerial Vehicles: Applications for Natural Resource Management and Monitoring." Paper presented at the 2004 Council on Forest Engineering (COFE) Conference "Machines and People, The Interface," Hot Springs, Arkansas, April 27–30.

Koehler, J., P. Thomson, and R. Hope. 2015. "Pump-Priming Payments for Sustainable Water Services in Rural Africa." *World Development* 74 (October): 397–411.

Koh, L. P., and S. A. Wich. 2012. "Dawn of Drone Ecology: Low-Cost Autonomous Aerial Vehicles for Conservation." *Tropical Conservation Science* 5 (2): 121–32.

Laliberte, A., J. E. Herrick, A. Rango, and C. Winters. 2010. "Acquisition, or Thorectification, and Object-Based Classification of Unmanned Aerial Vehicle (UAV) Imagery for Rangeland Monitoring." *Photogrammetric Engineering & Remote Sensing* 76 (6): 661–72.

McAllister, L. 2016. "We're Sensing a Change in Water Monitoring: Introducing the Arsenic Sensor Prize Competition." *The EPA Blog,* September 19. https://blog.epa .gov/blog/2016/09/were-sensing-a-change-in-water-monitoring-introducing-the -arsenic-sensor-prize-competition/.

Nagel, C. J. Beach, C. Iribagiza, and E. Thomas. 2015. "Evaluating the Cost Effectiveness of Cellular Instrumentation on Rural Handpumps to Improve Service Delivery—A Longitudinal Cohort Study in Rwanda." *Environmental Science and Technology* 49 (24): 14292–300.

Pearce, J., N. Dickinson, and K. Welle. 2015. "Technology, Data, and People: Opportunities and Pitfalls of Using ICT to Monitor Sustainable WASH Delivery." In *Infrastructure to Services: Trends in Monitoring Sustainable Water, Sanitation, and Hygiene Services* edited by Ton Schouten, Stef Smits, and John Butterworth. Rugby, U.K.: Practical Action Publishing.

Ram, P. 2010. "Practical Guidance for Measuring Handwashing Behavior." Water and Sanitation Working Paper, World Bank, Washington, DC.

Salamí, E., C. Barrado, and E. Pastor. 2014. "UAV Flight Experiments Applied to the Remote Sensing of Vegetated Areas." *Remote Sensing* 6 (11): 11051–81.

Sinha, A., C. L. Nagel, E. Thomas, W. P. Schmidt, B. Torondel, S. Boisson, and T. F. Clasen. 2016. "Assessing Latrine Use in Rural India: A Cross-Sectional Study Comparing

Reported Use and Passive Latrine Use Monitors." *American Journal of Tropical Medicine and Hygiene* 95 (3): 720–27.

Sobrino, J., J. C. Jiménez-Muñoz, and L. Paolini. 2004. "Land Surface Temperature Retrieval from LANDSAT TM 5." *Remote Sensing of Environment* 90 (4): 434–40.

Sorensen, J. P., D. J. Lapworth, B. P. Marchant, D. C. Nkhuwa, S. Pedley, M. E. Stuart, R. A. Bell, M. Chirwa, J. Kabika, M. Liemisa, and M. Chibesa. 2015. "In-Situ Tryptophan-like Fluorescence: A Real-Time Indicator of Faecal Contamination in Drinking Water Supplies." *Water Research* 81 (September): 38–46.

Thomas, E. A., and K. Mattson. 2013. "Instrumented Monitoring with Traditional Public Health Evaluation Methods: An Application to a Water, Sanitation and Hygiene Program in Jakarta, Indonesia." Mercy Corps, Portland, OR.

Thomas, E. S. Tellez-Sanchez, C. Wich, M. Kirby, L. Zambrano, G. Rosa, T. Clasen, and C. Nagel. 2016. "Behavioral Reactivity Associated with Electronic Monitoring of Environmental Health Interventions—A Cluster Randomized Trial with Water Filters and Cookstoves." *Environmental Science and Technology* 50 (7): 3773–80.

UNICEF (United Nations Children's Fund). 2014. *Real Time E. coli Detection*. New York, NY: UNICEF.

USAID (U.S. Agency for International Development). 2015. *Kenya Resilient Arid Lands Partnership for Integrated Development*. Washington, DC: USAID.

———. 2016. *USAID Launches 500 Million Birr Activity on World Water Day to Boost Ethiopia's One Wash National Program*. Washington, DC: USAID.

Weng, Q., D. Lu, and J. Schubring. 2004. "Estimation of Land Surface Temperature–Vegetation Abundance Relationship for Urban Heat Island Studies." *Remote Sensing of Environment* 89 (4): 467–83.

World Bank. 2017. *Nigeria WASH Poverty Diagnostic: Intermediate Review Meeting*. Washington, DC: World Bank Group.

Zarco-Tejada, P. J., R. Diaz-Varela, V. Angileri, and P. Loudjani. 2014. "Tree Height Quantification Using Very High Resolution Imagery Acquired from an Unmanned Aerial Vehicle (UAV) and Automatic 3D Photo-Reconstruction Methods." *European Journal of Agronomy* 55 (April): 89–99.

CHAPTER 6

Mobile, Cloud, and Big Data for Measuring Progress in WASH

Kwasi Boateng and Christina Barstow

Introduction

Efforts to assess the impact of water, sanitation, and hygiene (WASH) interventions often rely on data collected through person-to-person surveys, subjective observations, or expensive and time-consuming experimental studies. Data are ordinarily recorded by hand and processed on a per-project basis. These conventional approaches have limitations that affect the value of the derived data. With well-designed experimental studies such as randomized controlled trials, the data collected and subsequent impact analysis are often not available until well after the intervention is considered complete. This can delay providing input to subsequent interventions. Overarching these challenges is the bespoke nature of most data collection, analysis, and sharing systems that are either (i) inexpensive and limited or (ii) expensive and ample.

Technology-Based Tools for WASH Programs

Big data analytics and its attendant decision-making tools are poised to transform emerging and developing regions around the world and can help address these limitations of conventional data collection and action. The use of computing technology to track and measure water and sanitation quality and delivery is a rapidly growing field. Technology-based measurement methods can provide more repeatable results and increase accountability of sampling strategies. Much of technology-based monitoring of WASH has focused primarily on easier ways to collect and store data. The field of mobile surveys provides a user-friendly platform to easily collect data whereby the surveyor can insert data into a mobile form rather than using a paper-based survey. The mobile platform additionally allows for Global Positioning System (GPS) coordinates, barcode scanning, and photos to be easily associated with a particular sample. This creates both ease of data analysis and surveyor accountability thanks to quality control checks that can be realized by looking at photos of results or checking GPS coordinates for the correct location source. In this chapter, a number of electronic data collection and dissemination tools used in WASH programs are reviewed.

The Water Quality Reporter

The Water Quality Reporter (WQR) application was developed at the University of Cape Town as part of a consortium with several U.S. and U.K. organizations and academic institutions.[1] The WQR application uses Short Message Service (SMS) to report data with a cell phone. Because of the simplicity of SMS-based data collection, the application can be used on the most basic mobile phones. Users of the application submit water quality data such as chlorine residual testing or a presence–absence microbiological test. Near real-time reporting then allows for quick feedback mechanisms between water quality monitors and communities using the systems. Additionally the application is open source allowing for stakeholders at all levels to submit data (Labuschagne 2012).

mWater

The mWater platform is an open-source mobile survey application and data management tool to monitor water-related development programs while providing a collaborative space for sharing of data.[2] The services are free to use and the mobile app is fully functional offline, and thus can be applied in a variety of programs. Users develop mobile survey tools by means of the mWater portal, which is simple to use with basic training. mWater presently has over 17,000 unique users in 143 countries representing nonprofits, governments, and academic organizations. Nearly a million surveys have been collected for over 300,000 monitoring sites, which include water points, sanitation facilities, schools, and health facilities. mWater data can be restricted by organizations and users, or shared broadly with the public.

Originally conceived as a water quality–monitoring app, mWater has expanded to become a full-featured management information system for water and sanitation, also incorporating data from adjacent sectors such as health, education, and agriculture. Several countries now use mWater as their primary WASH sector–monitoring platform, including Guinea-Bissau (figure 6.1), Haiti, and Malawi. To support free users and increase the comparability of monitoring data, mWater developed a Global Indicator Library, organized by Sustainable Development Goal topics. Users can look up indicators by topic, read detailed documentation on their use, and then insert predefined question sets into their own survey forms. Through partnerships with WaterAid, the United Nations Children's Fund (UNICEF), and the World Health Organization, mWater has built core indicator sets for water point mapping, WASH in schools and health facilities, and water quality monitoring.

M-Maji

M-Maji uses feedback from water stakeholders via a simple mobile application to provide information on water availability, quality, and price.[3] Developed by researchers at Stanford University with partners in Kenya, the application

Figure 6.1 Example of mWater Dashboard for Water Point Monitoring

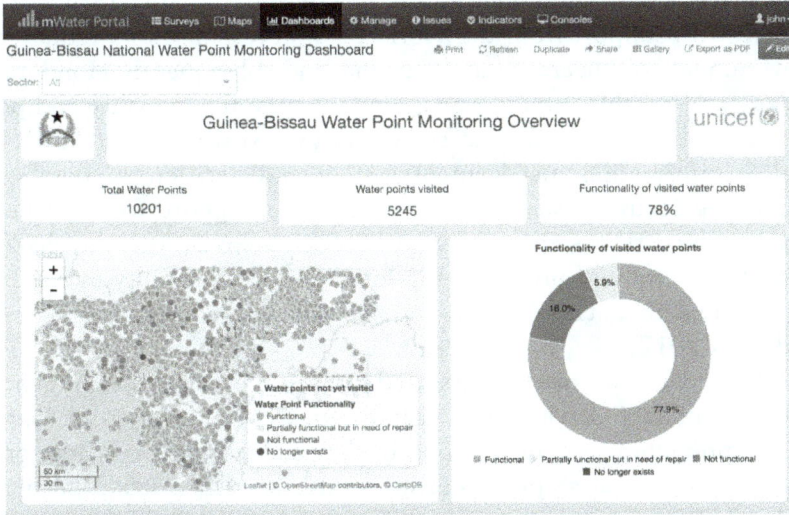

Source: mWater, http://www.mwater.co.

allows water vendors to advertise their water service and users to find their closest water points with information about the quality and price of the water. Water quality is specifically addressed through regular testing and spot checks of water points; a water source may be taken down or rated poorly if quality standards are not achieved. Additionally, users have the option to file a complaint, which may provide information on a source's changing water quality. M-Maji was implemented in Kibera, a slum in Kenya, where water is often contaminated, scarce, or expensive. Kibera households can spend large portions of their day trying to locate a water provider with an actual water supply, and then pay exorbitant prices for unsafe water. Use of M-Maji in Kibera has the potential to reduce costs from the purchase of water, reduce time spent searching for water, increase the quality of water consumed, and increase accountability of water providers.

The Portable Water Quality Field Kit

The Portable Water Quality Field Kit was developed by the WASH Monitoring, Evaluation and Learning center at the University of North Carolina.[4] Although similar to the idea of other water quality portable laboratories, the Portable Water Quality Field Kit includes a mobile phone and backup battery charger with samples barcoded to allow for rapid and easier data tracking. The kit also contains materials necessary for several chemical tests—including arsenic, fluoride, and chlorine—and uses the compartment bag test for microbiological testing. The kit has the capability to analyze dozens of samples with all materials contained in a portable backpack (Sobsey 2016).

The Rural Water and Sanitation Information System Initiative

The Rural Water and Sanitation Information System Initiative (SIASAR) was developed with support from the World Bank in response to a request from the governments of Nicaragua and Panama, and subsequently Honduras, for systematic and reliable information to monitor the functionality and performance of rural water supply and sanitation (WSS) services.[5] SIASAR is an innovative information management system and decision support system with a strong focus on sustainability. It aims to support a comprehensive approach to rural WSS service delivery. SIASAR helps address the challenges faced by the sector and promotes the long-term sustainability of rural WSS services by making data collection and analysis simpler and more accessible (World Bank 2017).

SIASAR's conceptual model is designed to assess the factors that influence the sustainability of WSS services over time through careful analysis of four core entities: communities, systems, service providers, and technical assistance providers. SIASAR's data analysis process involves three key steps: data collection and validation, indicator processing, and performance ranking. Field data pertaining to each entity are collected through a mobile application using four basic surveys. Once data are validated, a battery of indicators is automatically generated and aggregated into six thematic indexes (water service level, sanitation and hygiene service level, water system infrastructure, service provision, technical assistance provision, and WASH schools and health centers) that make up the Water and Sanitation Performance Index (WSP).

The information ecosystem supporting SIASAR consists of a suite of free, open-source, simple-yet-robust, modern information and communication technology (ICT) tools. It comprises a public website and a web-based user backend, multiplatform mobile applications, a data integration and business analytics engine, and a geo dashboard. SIASAR's flexible approach can respond to a context's specific requirements while ensuring data harmonization across scales to address the needs of different stakeholders enabling comparisons across space and time. The use of state-of-the-art technology to simplify data collection and processing renders SIASAR readily adaptable to future changes and requirements.

The unique collaborative and participatory process followed to develop this open system ensured the platform is driven by and tailored to the needs and characteristics of each participating member. In each country, the institution in charge of the rural WSS sector leads the implementation of SIASAR, is responsible for mainstreaming it through the sector institutional structure, and interacts with key actors involved across all levels. Government ownership and close collaboration with other donors and partners—such as the Swiss Agency for Development and Cooperation, the Spanish Agency for International Development Cooperation, the Inter-American Development Bank, the European Union, UNICEF, international nongovernmental organizations (NGOs), regional networks, and local organizations—have been key to SIASAR's consolidation and expansion.

Since its regional launch in Panama in July 2012, SIASAR has expanded to eight additional members, including Bolivia, Colombia, Costa Rica, Paraguay, Peru, the Brazilian State of Ceara, the Mexican State of Oaxaca, and the Dominican Republic. To date, the monitoring of more than 23,000 rural communities—with a total population of approximately 11 million people and covering approximately 19,500 water supply systems serviced by 17,500 service providers—has positively impacted rural users across the Latin America and Caribbean region. Underpinning its success is the initiative's commitment to eight Guiding Principles to create a product that is Simple, Robust, Institutionalized, Open, Harmonized, Adapted, Flexible, and Up-to-Date. SIASAR also seeks to promote transparency and social accountability by increasing visibility of the WSS sector at the community scale through its open access website.

Watertracker

New York–based company Arc Finance developed the community-centric reporting tool Watertracker for the Sustainable Water Supply and Sanitation project (SWSS) of the U.S. Agency for International Development (USAID) to help provide data on numerous water points in Afghan communities. Since 2009, USAID's SWSS mobilized Afghan residents to help in increasing access to safe drinking water and sanitation by building or renovating latrines and constructing water wells. Using the open-source platform UShahidi, Watertracker was used in monitoring and reporting information on close to 100,000 wells in Afghanistan through its Interactive Voice Response (IVR) platform. Watertracker's IVR service was able to store and map detailed information on thousands of water points in Afghanistan, and hundreds of reports led to the repair of several wells.

Akvo (FLOW, Really Simple Reporting, Lumen)

The Avko Foundation has several products used by over 1,000 organizations for managing water data.[6] FLOW is an open-source mapping software for mapping thousands of water points in far less time than traditional paper-based surveys would allow. It collects, evaluates, and displays large quantities of geographically referenced data using a smartphone app and an online dashboard, allowing situations on the ground to be mapped and changes to be monitored over time. This enables the use of accurate and current data in making informed investment decisions. Akvo Really Simple Reporting (RSR) serves as an online communication, reporting, and monitoring hub for projects. It allows the coordination of activities and monitoring of results in order to aid continuous improvement. The Akvo RSR offers program managers a structured stream of information and data pertaining to progress, results, and the flow of work. RSR further allows users to collect from and send information to other platforms, and hence pull data from RSR into other personal online systems. Akvo Lumen, a new dashboard tool, is designed to enable rapid and informative data visualization.

Jisomee Mita

This is a mobile-to-web platform that allows residents to submit water meter readings using SMS, check account numbers and water consumption balance, and pay their water bills. It was developed by the Nairobi City Water and Sewerage Company (NCWSC) as a way to empower consumers and increase revenue collection. Based on free, open-source technology, it allows NCWSC to cover the cost of sending responses to customers at a cheaper rate than issuing a paper bill.

MajiVoice

An initiative of Kenya's water sector regulator, the Water Services Regulatory Board, the MajiVoice platform promotes two-way communication between citizens and water service providers using SMS messages or the Internet.[7] It enables consumers to provide performance feedback while offering water service providers the ability to be more responsive to consumer needs and requirements. Furthermore, the use of georeferencing tools helps water service providers better understand the needs of different localities and identify areas that need improvement.

SeeSaw

SeeSaw is a South African social venture that combines ICT and WASH services, primarily focusing on technology and how well it is used.[8] SeeSaw designs and distributes software and consults for organizations by analyzing the particular context in which organizations operate and then offering software and advice customized for those organizations. For example, a survey developed by SeeSaw focuses on having a clear understanding of existing ICT tools pertaining to African water utilities, the demand for those tools, and overall market condition for those tools.

SeeSaw's technology (VerAgua), based on its SeeTell and SeeView platforms, uses the mobile services of free missed calls, SMS, and data to relay information about the status of water service. In order to file reports, caretakers are given laminated cards with unique phone numbers corresponding to specific water points. Caretakers then report on water status three days in a week, with the SeeTell web platform tracking all the calls in order to aggregate the status of all water points.

Service Level Benchmarking Connect

The WSP in consultation with India's Ministry of Urban Development started the Service Level Benchmarking Connect initiative in 2012 to provide a means of collecting feedback from citizens for integration into agencies' workflow. The feedback obtained, ranging from satisfaction levels to customers' services experiences, is compiled in a scorecard to enable interested stakeholders to measure the quality of services provided. In the future, Service Level Benchmarking Connect aims to integrate with state and national WASH programs in efforts to improve the tracking of service outcomes.

The Senegalaise des Eaux Supervision Cockpit

This is a modern call center with a computer platform supporting geolocations using GPS/GSM (Global System for Mobile Communications), a direct consultation inventory, and a computerized mapping system. The supervision cockpit aids in network efficiency in areas of reduced leakages, metering and billing improvements, and provision of a toll-free number that customers can use to lodge complaints and request other services. The Senegalaise des Eaux Supervision Cockpit has helped to increase network efficiency from 69 percent to 80 percent within 10 years.

The Water Point Data Exchange

The Water Point Data Exchange (WPDx)—released in May 2015 by the Global Water Challenge in partnership with businesses, NGOs, the World Bank, UNICEF, and World Vision—serves as a global platform for sharing water point data.[9] WPDx has aggregated data on about 250,000 water points in 25 countries from about 30 water sources. Data from different sources are collected and aggregated; any new data, whether on infrastructure or status update, are integrated into WPDx without overwriting the existing information, hence preserving a historical record of information. Data collected include location, date of information collection, water point type or source, and the presence or otherwise of water during the time of evaluation. Other sets of common indicators that could provide useful information may be collected in some cases. With better water data, it is expected that governments and NGOs will be able to allocate resources where they are most needed.

WASHCost Calculator

The San Francisco–based nonprofit organization WellDone International developed the WASHCost Calculator in response to the massive data and knowledge gap in the WASH sector, especially in remote and underserved areas.[10] The calculator performs budget calculations and sustainability checks for WASH programs and also serves as a forum for collecting critical cost data from donors, community organizations, and service providers. More data results in establishing better benchmarks in order to ensure smarter planning for organizations.

Water Point Mapper

The Water Point Mapper is a tool for producing maps indicating the status of water supply services.[11] Its target market is WASH practitioners and local governments at district and subdistrict levels in Sub-Saharan Africa. Developed by WaterAid, the Mapper provides a monitoring process for the distribution and status of water points in rural and urban areas and supports local-level planning for improving water sector performance accountability at local and national levels.

WaterWatchers

A 2011 census indicated that, although 93 percent of South African households had access to safe water in 2010, only 45 percent of those actually had water in their homes. Pressure on an ageing infrastructure and urban population influx are only two of the challenges facing water services provision and distribution. In response to some of these challenges, technology giant IBM sought to provide a single view of the issues by gathering an aggregate of vital data points for its "WaterWatchers" project. This project enabled citizens to report water leaks, faulty pipes, and other general conditions of water infrastructure via a mobile phone application and SMS capability. The data were then analyzed and aggregated after 30 days in order to generate a "leak hot spot" map for the country. The map subsequently enabled local municipalities, water control boards, water planners, and other water system stakeholders to visualize and prioritize improvements to water infrastructure across the country. By combining the concepts of big data, mobile technology, and crowdsourcing, IBM enabled cities in South Africa to better understand their water systems and undertake the needed improvements.

NextDrop

Many urban Indians, like their counterparts in other emerging economies, have mobile phones but not enough water. Even for those with water, it hardly gets to them in an efficient manner. In India's city of Hubbali, nearly one million people got water only every three to five days, and for just about four hours a day. The Indian start-up NextDrop, which began operations in 2010, devised a means by which it could address this problem: leveraging mobile text messages to create a water data system that could efficiently deliver water to consumers.[12] In conjunction with India's local government, the system sought to connect valve technicians to engineers and customers. NextDrop called valve technicians on a daily basis to obtain information on the level of water after the technicians had measured the level of water in reservoirs. The information was then subsequently sent to engineers to determine what areas needed water and in what quantity, depending on the available supply. NextDrop then sent texts to the valve technicians, which could subsequently be forwarded to customers to indicate when water would be released to them. This network provided much information that previously could not be easily gleaned by engineers, such as how much water was available, leaking pipes, and areas that got more water or areas that had been deprived of water. This information created some stability in an area where families were estimated to be spending some 20–40 hours per month scouting for water, and in some cases taking entire days off to collect water.

Challenges in Data Collection and Action

A key challenge in the WASH sector remains that of bringing together numerous stakeholders spanning different sectors while still using multitudes of data sets. Addressing this challenge requires ensuring the supply of high-quality data and improving analytical capacity by filling all WASH data gaps and strengthening data integration across multiple sectors. Furthermore, data applications stand the chance of helping governments in emerging economies address the myriad social and economic issues that continue to plague these regions. Opening up access to data and being more transparent on WASH sector projects may empower consumers to have more fruitful interactions with stakeholders. Creating proper dialogue with the use of big data applications is sure to provide both consumers and governments the proper tools required to address social and economic problems (Sullivan 2015).

Realizing these benefits requires proper coordination of the efforts of governments, development organizations, and the private sector through the creation of a conducive environment for sharing mobile-generated data. Government policies and legal frameworks should adequately protect individuals and corporate entities alike, and development organizations' support needs to constantly demonstrate the public good that big data seek to offer.

Notes

1. For more information about the WQR application, see the Imagination for People website, http://imaginationforpeople.org/en/project/the-water-quality-reporter-wqr -application/.

2. For more information about mWater, see the company's website, http://www .mwater.co.

3. For more information about the M-Maji application, see M-Maji's website, https:// mmaji.wordpress.com.

4. For more information on the Portable Water Quality Field Kit, see the Aquagenx website, https://www.aquagenx.com.

5. More information on the initiative is available on SIASAR's website, http://www .siasar.org/en.

6. Information in the section comes from the Akvo website. For more information, see https://akvo.org.

7. For more information on MajiVoice, see the company's website, http://www .majivoice.com.

8. More information on SeeSaw is available from the company's website, http://www .greenseesaw.com/.

9. For more information on the exchange, see the Water Point website, https://www .waterpointdata.org.

10. For more information on the WASHCost Calculator, see the organization's website, http://www.ircwash.org/washcost.

11. More information on the Water Point Mapper and other water mapping tools is available at http://www.waterpointmapper.org.

12. For more information, see NextDrop's website, https://nextdrop.co.

References

Labuschagne, L. 2012. "Water Monitoring 'Easier' with Free Mobile Phone App." *SciDev. Net*, March 30. http://www.scidev.net/global/r-d/news/water-monitoring-easier-with -free-mobile-phone-app.html.

Sobsey, M. D. 2016. "Why Test Drinking and Other Waters?" From the World Bank webinar "Water Quality Testing: Everything You Always Wanted to Know," Washington, DC, October 5.

Sullivan, M. 2015. "Turning Citizens into Sensors: Using Mobile Apps and 'Big Data' to Combat Water Losses in South Africa." *Water & Sanitation for the Urban Poor* (blog), June 3. http://www.wsup.com/2015/06/03/turning-citizens-into-sensors-using-mobile -apps-and-big-data-to-combat-water-losses-in-south-africa/.

World Bank. 2017. *Consolidation, Improvement and Expansion of the Rural Water and Sanitation Information System (SIASAR)*. Washington, DC: World Bank.

Household Surveys within WASH Monitoring Indicators

Libbet Loughnan

Introduction

The water, sanitation, and hygiene (WASH) framework of the Millenium Development Goals (MDGs) relied primarily on measurements collected through household surveys. That monitoring will be built into the Sustainable Development Goals (SDGs) monitoring, supplemented with evidence from other sources. The main classifications under the SDG monitoring time frame can be seen in figures A.1, A.2, and A.3. As such, the institutional knowledge, efforts, and successes built and achieved under the MDG time frame remain relevant and contribute building blocks of SDG monitoring. This appendix begins by laying out the long-collected measurements used in MDG monitoring. Their continued collection remains fundamental for future monitoring under the SDGs. Second, this appendix specifies how other measurements collected during the MDG time frame but not critical to MDG monitoring now make their way formally into SDG monitoring. These first two groups of measurements can be understood to meet all eight criteria for indicator selection and data sources listed in chapter 1. Third, the category of household survey–based measurements that are critical to SDG monitoring but that are only recently being rolled out for widespread collection will be outlined. All these elements of SDG monitoring that come from household surveys are noted in chapter 1, table 1.1, as "can be reported immediately" or "can be reported in the short term" because the technology is fully ready and either widespread historically or being rolled out. Last, the appendix closes with a review of some main challenges and opportunities in the full rollout of these household survey components of SDG measurements.

Long-Standing Household Survey–Based Measurements, Critical in Both MDG and SDG Monitoring

The measurements that MDG WASH assessments relied on were all self-reported by households and have been retained in the SDG time frame.

Figure A.1 The Rungs of the SDG Drinking Water Monitoring Ladder

Drinking Water Ladder

Safely managed
Drinking water from an improved water source which is located on premises,
available when needed, and free of faecal and priority contamination

Basic
Drinking water from an improved source, provided collection time is not more than
30 minutes for a round trip, including queuing

Limited
Drinking water from an improved source where collection time exceeds
30 minutes for a round trip to collect water, including queuing

Unimproved
Drinking water from an unprotected dug well or unprotected spring

Surface water
Drinking water directly from a river, dam, lake, pond, stream, canal, or irrigation
channel

Source: WHO/UNICEF 2017.
Note: SDG = Sustainable Development Goal.

Figure A.2 The Rungs of the SDG Sanitation Monitoring Ladder

Sanitation Ladder

Safely managed
Use of an improved sanitation facility that is not shared with other households and
where excreta are safely disposed in situ or transported and treated off-site

Basic
Use of improved facilities that are not shared with other households

Limited
Use of improved facilities shared between two or more households

Unimproved
Use of pit latrines without a slab or platform, hanging latrines, and bucket latrines

Open defecation
Disposal of human faeces in fields, forest, bushes, open bodies of water, beaches, or
other open spaces or with solid waste

Source: WHO/UNICEF 2017.
Note: SDG = Sustainable Development Goal.

Water

As mentioned in chapter 1, the proposed indicator of "safely managed drinking
water services" comprises four subelements, all of which rely on household
surveys: (i) an "improved drinking water source," which is (ii) "located on
premises," (ii) "available when needed," and (iv) "compliant with fecal

Figure A.3 The Rungs of the SDG Handwashing Monitoring Ladder

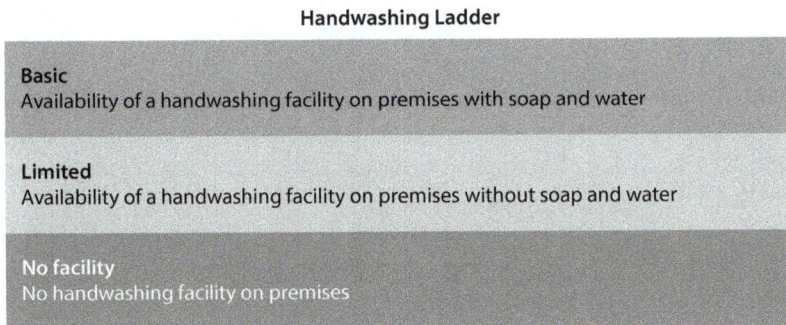

Handwashing Ladder

Basic Availability of a handwashing facility on premises with soap and water
Limited Availability of a handwashing facility on premises without soap and water
No facility No handwashing facility on premises

Source: WHO/UNICEF 2017.
Note: SDG = Sustainable Development Goal.

(and priority chemical) standards" (figure A.1). Of these, information on whether a household primarily uses an improved drinking water source has long been collected and was the main measurement used throughout MDG monitoring (see table A.1). This remains the recommendation for how a country collects the information for SDG monitoring, and means that the measurement offers one of the necessary criteria of "safely managed." It also allows delineation between "limited," "unimproved," and "surface water." If the country has strong seasonality, information on the differences between seasons would be collected, too.

Sanitation
The proposed indicator of "safely managed sanitation services" relies on household surveys for verification that the population of interest is using (i) an "improved type of sanitation facility," which is (ii) "not shared with other households," as well as for some of the relevant information for understanding (iii) whether the "excreta is safely disposed in situ." Of the five rungs in the Joint Monitoring Programme (JMP)'s ladder for monitoring progress in sanitation under the SDGs (see figure A.2), outlined in the other chapters, these measurements allow delineation between "limited" and "basic," and go part way to defining the relevant segment with "safely managed" sanitation among the population of interest. Of these three elements, the first two have long been collected and were the main measurements used throughout MDG monitoring (see table A.2).

The Progressive Reduction of Inequality
During the MDG time frame, monitoring was calculated separately for urban and rural segments of the population. This background characteristic will continue to be used in monitoring to examine whether the progressive reduction of inequality is being upheld. In addition, the calculation of subcategories of

Table A.1 MDG Household Survey Drinking Water Questions Retained for SDG Monitoring

WS1. What is the main source of drinking water used by members of your household?	**Piped water**	
	Piped into dwelling-------------------- 11	11⇨WS7
WS2. What is the main source of drinking water used by members of your household for other purposes, such as cooking and handwashing?[a]	Piped to yard/plot --------------------- 12	12⇨WS7
	Piped to neighbor --------------------- 13	13⇨WS3
	Public tap/standpipe------------------ 14	14⇨WS3
If unclear, probe to identify the place from which members of this household most often collect drinking water (collection point).	Tube well/borehole---------------------- 21	21⇨WS3
	Dug well	
	Protected well--------------------------31	31⇨WS3
	Unprotected well ----------------------32	32⇨WS3
	Spring	
	Protected spring ----------------------- 41	41⇨WS3
	Unprotected spring ------------------- 42	42⇨WS3
	Rainwater----------------------------------- 51	51⇨WS3
	Tanker-truck -------------------------------61	61⇨WS4
	Cart with small tank ---------------------- 71	71⇨WS4
	Water kiosk----------------------------------- 72	72⇨WS4
	Surface water (river, dam, lake, pond, stream, canal, irrigation channel) ----- 81	81⇨WS3
	Packaged water	
	Bottled water---------------------------- 91	
	Sachet water --------------------------- 92	
	Other (*specify*) ----------------------------- 96	96⇨WS3

Source: MICS6 Household Questionnaire, November 2017 version (check http://mics.unicef.org/tools?round=mics6 for updates).
Note: MDG = Millenium Development Goal; SDG = Sustainable Development Goal; WS = survey module code standing for "water and sanitation."
a. Same responses as WS1, skips the same except for packaged water, which goes to WS4.

Table A.2 MDG Household Survey Sanitation Monitoring Questions Retained for SDG Monitoring

WS11. What kind of toilet facility do members of your household usually use?	**Flush/pour flush**	
	Flush to piped sewer system ----------- 11	11⇨WS14
	Flush to septic tank-------------------- 12	
If "Flush" or "Pour flush," probe:	Flush to pit latrine--------------------- 13	
Where does it flush to?	Flush to open drain-------------------- 14	14⇨WS14
	Flush to DK where --------------------- 18	18⇨WS14
If not possible to determine, ask permission to observe the facility.	**Pit latrine**	
	Ventilated improved pit latrine--------------------------------------- 21	
	Pit latrine with slab ------------------- 22	
	Pit latrine without slab/ Open pit--------------------------------- 23	
	Composting toilet------------------------ 31	
	Bucket --------------------------------------- 41	41⇨WS14

table continues next page

Table A.2 MDG Household Survey Sanitation Monitoring Questions Retained for SDG Monitoring *(continued)*

	Hanging toilet/		
	Hanging latrine ------------------------- 51	51⇨WS14	
	No facility/bush/field --------------------- 95	95⇨*End*	
	Other *(specify)* ---------------------------- 96	96⇨WS14	
WS14. Where is this toilet facility located?	In own dwelling--------------------------- 1		
	In own yard/plot-------------------------- 2		
	Elsewhere----------------------------------- 3		
WS15. Do you share this facility with others who are not members of your household?	Yes -- 1		
	No-- 2	2⇨*End*	

Source: MICS6 Household Questionnaire, November 2017 version (check http://mics.unicef.org/tools?round=mics6 for updates).
Note: MDG = Millenium Development Goal; SDG = Sustainable Development Goal; WS = survey module code standing for "water and sanitation."

access and lack of access, and their differing severities represented by ranking in "ladder" rungs, will continue during the SDG time frame, and will help quantify inequities.

Long-Standing Household Survey–Based Measurements, Not Used in MDG Monitoring but Critical for SDG Monitoring

Water

Household surveys are the recommended tool through which a country can verify that the improved drinking water source is "within 30 minutes roundtrip," and "located on premises" (see table A.3).

These recommended survey questions were rolled out widely during the MDG period, partially because of efforts by the Multiple Indicator Cluster Surveys (MICS), Demographic and Health Surveys (DHS), and other survey teams, to support international recommendations led by the JMP. The information collected under it was regularly used by the JMP, but not as a critical input to the MDG assessment of access to improved drinking water. Inferences on "available when needed" can also be made from this measurement until the new measurement outlined below can be rolled out. Hence, these measurements allow delineation between "basic" and "limited," as well as contributing the "on premises" verification needed as part of the delineation between "safely managed" and "basic," in the ladder for monitoring progress in drinking water under the SDGs.

Hygiene

The hygiene element of the SDGs also relies fully on the continued collection of measurements that have long been collected through household surveys, but which were not monitored under regular MDG reporting (see figure A.3). As core measurements in the MICS and DHS since 2009, data availability is already widespread. Alongside data self-reported by households, this measurement extends the group of SDG WASH measurements relying on household survey data to observation-based measurement. These measurements

Table A.3 Long-Standing Household Survey Water Questions Newly Critical under SDG Monitoring

WS3. Where is that water source located?	In own dwelling---------------------------- 1	1⇨WS7
	In own yard/plot-------------------------- 2	2⇨WS7
	Elsewhere----------------------------------- 3	
WS4. How long does it take for members of your household to go there, get water, and come back?	Members do not collect ----------------- 000 Number of minutes --------------------- DK-- 998	000 ⇨WS7

Source: MICS6 Household Questionnaire, November 2017 version (check http://mics.unicef.org/tools?round=mics6 for updates).
Note: DK = don't know; SDG = Sustainable Development Goal; WS = a survey module code standing for "water and sanitation."

Table A.4 Long-Standing Household Survey Handwashing Measurements Newly Critical under SDG Monitoring

HW1. We would like to learn about where members of this household wash their hands.
 	
Can you please show me where members of your household most often wash their hands?
 	
Record result and observation.
	Observed
	Fixed facility observed (sink/tap)
	   In dwelling------------------------------ 1
	   In yard/plot----------------------------- 2
	Mobile object observed
	   (Bucket/jug/kettle) -------------------- 3
	
	Not observed
	No hand washing place in dwelling/
	   Yard/plot --------------------------------- 4
	No permission to see--------------------- 5
	Other reason (*specify* --------------------- 6
		4⇨*HW5*
		5⇨*HW4*
		6⇨*HW5*

HW2. *Observe presence of water at the place for handwashing.* *Verify by checking the tap/pump, or basin, bucket, water container or similar objects for presence of water.*	Water is available------------------------- 1 Water is not available--------------------- 2	
HW3. *Is soap or detergent present at the place for handwashing?*	Yes, present --------------------------------- 1 No, not present ------------------------------ 2	1⇨*HW7* 2⇨*HW5*

Source: MICS6 Household Questionnaire, November 2017 version (check http://mics.unicef.org/tools?round=mics6 for updates).
Note: HW = survey module code standing for "handwashing"; SDG = Sustainable Development Goal.

allow delineation between all three classifications in the ladder for monitoring progress in hygiene under the SDGs (see figure A.3 and table A.4).

The Progressive Reduction of Inequality

Additional background characteristics already widely collected in household surveys and censuses can be put to new use to examine whether the progressive reduction of inequality is being upheld. Examples among them include religion, ethnicity, geographic location, and wealth or income status. In addition, although not critical to official MDG monitoring, the following measurements presented in tables A.5 and A.6 were increasingly used and are now critically relevant to

Table A.5 Long-Standing Household Survey Drinking Water Questions Relevant for SDG Monitoring of Equality

WS5. Who usually goes to this source to collect the water for your household?	Name _____
Record the name of the person and copy the line number of this person from the LIST OF HOUSEHOLD MEMBERS Module.	Line number ------------------------------- ⎯⎯
WS6. Since last (**day of the week**), how many times has this person collected water?	Number of times ------------------------- ⎯⎯ DK--- 98

Source: MICS6 Household Questionnaire, November 2017 version (check http://mics.unicef.org/tools?round=mics6 for updates).
Note: DK = don't know; SDG = Sustainable Development Goal; WS = a survey module code standing for "water and sanitation."

Table A.6 Long-Standing Household Survey Sanitation Questions Relevant for SDG Monitoring of Equality

CA30. *Check* UB2: *Child's age?*	Age 0, 1 or 2--------------------------------- 1	
	Age 3 or 4------------------------------------ 2	2⇨*End*
CA31. The last time (*name*) passed stools, what was done to dispose of the stools?	Child used toilet/latrine ------------------ 01	
	Put/rinsed into toilet	
	or latrine -------------------------------- 02	
	Put/rinsed into drain or ditch ---------- 03	
	Thrown into garbage	
	(solid waste)----------------------------- 04	
	Buried--- 05	
	Left in the open --------------------------- 06	
	Other (*specify*) _____ 96	
	DK--- 98	

Source: MICS6 Questionnaire for Children Under Five, November 2017 version (check http://mics.unicef.org/tools?round=mics6 for updates).
Note: CA = survey module code standing for "care of illness"; DK = don't know; SDG = Sustainable Development Goal; UB = survey module code standing for "under-five's background."

monitoring the progressive reduction of intergenerational, intrahousehold, or gender dimensions of inequities.

Additional gender dimensions can be inferred from measurements noted above on open defecation and access to handwashing materials.

Household Survey Measurements Now Being Collected

Water

The testing of whether there is zero *Escherichia coli* in 100 mL of a household's drinking water should be rolled out in household surveys as soon as resources allow because it is critical for determining a baseline against which to prioritize action and verify success. The testing is a critical component in enabling delineation between "safely managed" and "limited" in the JMP's ladder for monitoring progress in drinking water under the SDGs. The template survey elements for this are not all listed here, but they can be found on the JMP website; and chapter 1 of this book examines this measurement in further detail.

Table A.7 Newer Household Survey Drinking Water Question Critical under SDG Monitoring

WS7. In the last month, has there been any time when your household did not have sufficient quantities of drinking water?	Yes, at least once--------------------------- 1	
	No, always sufficient ---------------------- 2	2⇨WS9
	DK--- 8	8⇨WS9

Source: MICS6 Household Questionnaire, November 2017 version (check http://mics.unicef.org/tools?round=mics6 for updates).
Note: DK = don't know; SDG = Sustainable Development Goal; WS = survey module standing for "water and sanitation."

Table A.8 Newer Household Survey Sanitation Questions Critical under SDG Monitoring

WS12. Has your (*answer from WS11*) ever been emptied?	Yes, emptied	
	Within the last 5 years --------------- 1	
	More than 5 years ago --------------- 2	
	Don't know when -------------------- 3	
	No, never emptied ---------------------- 4	4⇨WS14
	DK--- 8	8⇨WS14
WS13. The last time it was emptied, where were the contents emptied to? *Probe:* Was it removed by a service provider?	**Removed by service provider**	
	To a treatment plant ------------------ 1	
	Buried in a covered pit --------------- 2	
	To don't know where ----------------- 3	
	Emptied by household	
	Buried in a covered pit --------------- 4	
	To uncovered pit, open ground, water body or elsewhere ------------ 5	
	Other (*specify*) _____ 6	
	DK--- 8	

Source: MICS6 Household Questionnaire, November 2017 version (check http://mics.unicef.org/tools?round=mics6 for updates).
Note: DK = don't know; SDG = Sustainable Development Goal; WS = survey module standing for "water and sanitation."

The recommended measurement on "available when needed" (see table A.7) can contribute the "available when needed" verification as part of the delineation between "safely managed" and "basic," in the ladder for monitoring progress in drinking water under the SDGs.

Sanitation

The newly used measurement presented in table A.8 is amenable for full and rapid rollout in household surveys in the sense that it involves just one self-reported measurement. It goes as far as a household survey can for contributing to delineating "safely managed" sanitation.

The Progressive Reduction of Inequality

Table A.9 presents questions that are being widely rolled out and can help contribute to examining whether gender and sex biases exist in WASH.

It is likely that over time additional measurements from household surveys will be used to help support a countries' planning for efficiently and effectively reducing inequity and working toward universal access.

Table A.9 Newer Household Survey Hygiene Questions Increasingly Relevant for Monitoring Equality

UN16. Due to your last menstruation, were there any social activities or school or work days that you did not attend?	Yes --1 No---2 DK/not sure/no such activity------------------------8
UN17. During your last menstrual period were you able to wash and change in privacy while at home?	Yes --1 No---2 DK---8

Source: MICS6 Questionnaire for Individual Women, November 2017 version (check http://mics.unicef.org/tools?round=mics6 for updates).
Note: These questions should only be asked of women who have had a period in the preceding year and must be asked in private. They are typically asked as part of the women's questionnaire in the context of unmet health needs. DK = don't know; SDG = Sustainable Development Goal; UN = survey module code standing for "unmet need."

Recommendations and Opportunities for Optimizing the Collection of Household Survey Measurements

This increase in the range of measurements from household surveys that will be built into SDG monitoring represents challenges. Along with new straightforward questions that collect data through a household's self-reported response, the surveys involve more training and resource-intensive observation-based measurements and direct water quality testing. Achieving this will be a major task: despite the JMP's advocacy and engagement with countries throughout the MDG period, even in 2015 some countries had not yet collected good data.

The following categories of action can help ensure strategic use of the limited resources that are available for collecting SDG WASH data through household surveys:

- Broad dissemination of information on the measurements
- Identification of data gaps
- Ranking, prioritization, and strategizing for address

Within the global community, the following actors have perhaps the greatest opportunities and responsibilities, and can gain the greatest benefits from working together on these activities: the designated monitoring agency—the JMP—along with international stakeholders such as the World Bank, countries, and the populations without access. All have relevant contributions to this conversation.

It is worth noting that each stakeholder logically has a unique mix of competing incentives that must be borne in mind and responsibly managed. These include the need to develop valid, reliable, and impartial evidence; fill data gaps; streamline reporting; verify any success, and so on.

The World Bank, JMP and many of the national actors are already working on these activities, but massive efficiencies can be gained. Specific recommended examples of action under each activity include but are not limited to the following:

- **Broad dissemination of information on the measurements**, so that the first opportunity for rollout can be taken. Here the JMP and international actors such as the World Bank have the greatest opportunities. Although the SDG monitoring framework is based on bottom-up contributions in a degree unprecedented during the MDGs, ultimately the ratified structure needs to be communicated back from centralized levels to all stakeholders. The JMP is widely disseminating a set of reports on this, and teams in the World Bank, such as the WASH Poverty Diagnostics, are furthering this dissemination. One planned element that will greatly aid this work is the JMP's release of an updated "Core WASH Measurements for Household Surveys," the last version of which was released in 2006. The World Bank is meanwhile housing a living document to bridge the gap.
- **Identification of data gaps against each necessary measurement** should include, for example, quantification in terms of percentage and number of the relevant population. The JMP's monitoring products—such as its "country files"—can readily be used as inputs. Resources would have to be dedicated for purposeful extraction of the relevant information from their calculations. In the WASH Poverty Diagnostics countries, the JMP and World Bank already partner in work along these lines.
- **Ranking, prioritization, and strategizing for address**. Anticipated considerations include whether the gaps are long-standing, the resource intensity involved in their collection, severity of the issue, perceived relevance of issue resolution for national monitoring priorities, and so on. Cooperation between international survey agencies (for example, the Living Standards Measurement Study, DHS, and MICS, including in official memorandums of understanding), is being furthered to support this. An example of extensive partnership work can be seen from Ecuador, where the main MDG data gaps were largely resolved in a single survey in December of 2016, and the SDG baseline collected.

References

UNICEF. 2017. MICS6 Household Questionnaires (MICS6 Household Questionnaire, MICS6 Questionnaire for Individual Women, and MICS6 Questionnaire for Children under Five). Accessed November 29, 2017, at http://mics.unicef.org/tools?round=mics6.

WHO/UNICEF (World Health Organization/United Nations Children's Fund Joint Monitoring Programme for Water, Sanitation, and Hygiene). 2017. Monitoring pages. Accessed November 29, 2017, at https://washdata.org/monitoring.

Technologies and Data-Sharing Platforms for WASH Data

Table B.1 Technologies and Data-Sharing Platforms for WASH Data

Technology/Platform	Summary	Developers/Stakeholders	Launch year	Countries	Links
Akvo (Really Simple Reporting, RSR)	Online communication, reporting, and monitoring hub for projects. Allows coordination of activities and monitoring of results to promote continuous improvement.	Akvo	2008	Worldwide	http://akvo.org/products/rsr/#overview
Akvo (FLOW, OpenAid)	Multilanguage tool for collecting and displaying geographically referenced data.	Akvo	2010	Africa, Asia, and Americas	http://akvo.org/products/akvoflow/
International Aid Transparency Initiative	A framework for publishing data on development cooperation activities to serve all organizations involved in development, such as government sector organizations, national and international NGOs.	A variety of international donors, governments, and NGOs	2008	Worldwide	http://www.aidtransparency.net/
Taarifa	An open-source web application allowing public officials to respond to citizen complaints about sanitation delivery services.	Bill and Melinda Gates Foundation, Nokia, Toilet Hackers, Taarifa	2011	Tanzania, Uganda, Ghana	www.taarifa.org
The Water Point Data Exchange	A global platform for sharing water point data by aggregating data on thousands of water points from different water sources in different countries.	Global Water Challenge, the World Bank, UNICEF, World Vision, number of businesses, and NGOs	2015	Worldwide	https://www.waterpointdata.org
The Senegalaise des Eaux (SDE) Supervision Cockpit	A modern call center with a computer platform supporting geolocations using GPS/GSM, a direct consultation inventory, and a computerized mapping system for network efficiency, metering, and billing improvements.	Government of Senegal	2004	Senegal	http://www.sde.sn/Pages/accueil.aspx

table continues next page

Table B.1 Technologies and Data-Sharing Platforms for WASH Data *(continued)*

Technology/Platform	Summary	Developers/Stakeholders	Launch year	Countries	Links
WASHCost calculator	A tool for performing budget calculations and sustainability checks for WASH programs and for collecting critical cost data from donors, community organizations, and service providers.	WellDone International, IRC	2013	Worldwide	http://www.ircwash.org/blog /what-can-wash-cost -calculator-do-you-jim-yoon -welldone
Water Point Mapper	A tool for producing maps indicating water supply points and their status.	WaterAid	2011	Sub-Saharan Africa	http://www.waterpointmapper .org/
MajiData	Online database that assists water service providers and water service boards in preparing tailor-made proposals for urban slums and low-income areas within their service areas.	Kenya's Ministry of Water and Irrigation (MWI) and the Water Services Trust Fund (WSTF)	2011	Kenya	http://www.majidata.go.ke/
WaterTracker (Tetra Tech, Afghanistan)	A community-centric reporting tool for monitoring water points throughout Afghanistan. Codes assigned to new wells and community members can call to report broken wells in order to have them fixed.	Arc Finance, Tetra Tech, USAID	2012	Afghanistan	https://www.usaid.gov/global -waters/june-2012/starts -with-sustainability
WATEX	A groundwater exploration package for locating renewable ground water reserves in arid and semi-arid environments.	RTI, UNESCO, UNICEF	2004, 2006, 2013	Kenya, Chad, Sudan	www.rtiexploration.com/water/
Sanipath Rapid Assessment Tool		Rollins School of Public Health, Emory University	2014	Ghana, India, Mozambique	http://sanipath.org/

table continues next page

Table B.1 Technologies and Data-Sharing Platforms for WASH Data (continued)

Technology/Platform	Summary	Developers/Stakeholders	Launch year	Countries	Links
OpenDataKit	Free, open-source tool to author, field, and manage mobile data collection	University of Washington Computer Science and Engineering	2008	Worldwide	https://opendatakit.org/
DropDrop	Mobile app that allows users to track their water consumption with access to daily water usage reports and estimated water bills.	iCOMMS (University of Cape Town), City of Cape Town	2013	South Africa	http://www.icomms.uct.ac.za /dropdrop_icomms
Human Sensor Web (H2O)	Community-driven services for focused and georeferenced monitoring of water supply and sanitation coverage, that allows users to report water point failures	UN Habitat, google.org, GTZ Kenya, Water Services Trust Fund Kenya, WaterAid, Zantel, Zanzibar Water Authority, Upande, iNet/ Zanzibar Datacom Ltd.	2008–2010	Tanzania	http://52north.org/resources /references/sensor-web/h20
Jisomee Mita	Mobile to web platform that allows residents to submit water meter readings via SMS, check account numbers and water consumption balance, and make water bill payments	Nairobi City Water and Sewerage Company, WSP of the World Bank	2014	Kenya	http://nwater.jambopay.co.ke /accountcheck.php
M4W (Mobiles for Water)	SMS messages web interfaces are used to collect water and sanitation sector information and data are uploaded and hosted on the Internet for access by all relevant stakeholders.	Makerere University	2011	Uganda	http://m4water.org/

table continues next page

Table B.1 Technologies and Data-Sharing Platforms for WASH Data *(continued)*

Technology/Platform	Summary	Developers/Stakeholders	Launch year	Countries	Links
MajiMatone	A mobile-enabled technology that allows citizens to hold local government accountable for their rural water supplies in fixing broken down water points and services	DfID, Twaweza, Daraja and District Water Engineers	2010–2011	Tanzania	http://www.daraja.org
MajiVoice	An application used to improve communication between citizens and the Nairobi City Water and Sewerage Company	The World Bank, Nairobi City Water and Sewerage Company	2013	Kenya	http://www.majivoice.com
M-Maji	A mobile application for improving clean water access in slums through provision of water availability, price, and quality information by vendors	Stanford University, Umande Trust	2013	Kenya, Nairobi	https://mmaji.wordpress.com/
Mobile field assistant	A mobile meter reader with meter reading functions	Nairobi City Water and Sewerage Company	2014	Kenya	http://www.nairobiwater.co.ke
NextDrop	An SMS-based software product that allows citizens to be informed about water issues such as when they will get water, delays in supply, and damages that affect water supply.	Gates Foundation, UC Berkeley, Deshpande Foundation, Karnataka Water Board, Hubli-Dharwad Municipal Corporation (HDMC)	2010	India	www.nextdrop.org
SeeSaw	A social venture that combines ICT and WASH services with a primary focus on not just the technology but how it is used, by designing specific solutions for organizations based on their operations	SeeSaw, South Africa	2011	Southern Africa, West Africa, East and Central Africa, Other parts of the world	http://www.greenseesaw.com/

table continues next page

97

Table B.1 Technologies and Data-Sharing Platforms for WASH Data *(continued)*

Technology/Platform	Summary	Developers/Stakeholders	Launch year	Countries	Links
Service Level Benchmarking (SLB) Connect	A system for collection of citizens' feedback for integration into agencies' workflow in order to measure service quality and improve tracking of service outcomes	Ministry of Urban Development, India and the World Bank	2012	India	https://www.wsp.org /FeaturesEvents/Features /using-technology-track-how -citizens-experience-water -service-delivery-india
NFC RFID-Tracked Drinking Water	Programmed near-field communication phones with RFID used by Haitian water technicians in tracking chlorine usage in thousands of households.	Deep Springs International, Nokia Research Center, Palo Alto and UC Berkeley	2011	Haiti	http://www.nfcworld .com/2011/03/11/36414/nfc -phones-help-provide-clean -water-to-haitiearthquake -victims/
Smart hand pumps	SIM-card fitted hand pumps that provide low-cost automated real-time monitoring of hand pump functionality	Oxford University	2011	Kenya, Zambia	http://oxwater.co.uk/#/smart -handpumps/4559322273
Smart water metering	A system that measures detailed water consumption or abstraction and relays the information for monitoring and billing purposes	DfID	2002	Kenya, Zambia	http://r4d.dfid.gov.uk/PDF /Outputs/Water/
Water Quality Reporter	A low-cost, sustainable water test for monitoring drinking water quality and water sources critical to delivery of safe drinking water	iCOMMS, University of Bristol, Aquaya Institute of Health, Health Protection Agency, University of Cape Town, PATH, UC Berkeley, University of North Carolina, University of Southampton, University of Surrey, European Union, Bill and Melinda Gates Foundation	2009	South Africa, Mozambique, Vietnam and Cambodia	www.icomms.uct.ac.za/about _aquatest

table continues next page

Table B.1 Technologies and Data-Sharing Platforms for WASH Data *(continued)*

Technology/Platform	Summary	Developers/Stakeholders	Launch year	Countries	Links
Passive Latrine Use Monitors (PLUMs)	A low-cost motion sensor for monitoring latrine use	Portland State/SweetSense Inc.	2014	Kenya, India, Bangladesh, Indonesia	http://www.sweetsensors.com/
Water filter use	Sensors attached to the LifeStraw Family 1.0, 2.0 and the Unilever PureIt monitor use and water volume.	Portland State/SweetSense Inc.	2014	Rwanda, Kenya	http://www.sweetsensors.com/
CellPump	Cellular and satellite sensors for monitoring hand pumps including the AfriDev, India Mark 2, and Consellen	Portland State/SweetSense Inc.	2014	Rwanda, Uganda, Kenya	http://www.sweetsensors.com/
Borehole sensors	Cellular and satellite sensors to monitor functionality and service delivery at powered borehole sites	Portland State/SweetSense Inc.	2015	Ethiopia, Kenya	http://www.sweetsensors.com/
SmartSoap	An accelerometer placed within an ordinary-looking bar of soap that measures motion on three axes to estimate the number of handwashing events	Lifebuoy—Unilever	2009	Bangladesh, India	https://www.unilever.com/Images/lifebuoy-way-of-life_2010-12-oct12_tcm13-355913_tcm244-409755_en.pdf
Defecation motion sensor	An accelerometer placed on a water container used exclusively for anal cleansing that can be used to estimate the number of defecation events	Lifebuoy—Unilever	2009	India	Use of Electronic Loggers to Measure Changes in the Rates of Hand Washing with Soap in Low-Income Urban Households in India http://journals.plos.org/plosone/article?id=10.1371/journal.pone.0131187

table continues next page

Table B.1 Technologies and Data-Sharing Platforms for WASH Data *(continued)*

Technology/Platform	Summary	Developers/Stakeholders	Launch year	Countries	Links
Video observation	Video observation of handwashing practice	Various	2008	Kenya, New York, various	https://news.stanford.edu/news/2014/april/watching-hand-washing-041414.html
Akvo Caddisfly	A low-cost, open-source, smartphone-based drinking water testing system connected to an online data platform.	Akvo	2017	Africa, Asia, and Europe	http://akvo.org/akvo-caddisfly/
Color-changing handwash	Changing color of the foam shows that children have washed their hands long enough to remove germs.	Lifebuoy—Unilever	2012	India	https://www.unilever.com/sustainable-living/the-sustainable-living-plan/improving-health-and-well-being/health-and-hygiene/changing-hygiene-habits-for-better-health/innovation-for-handwashing.html
Soap and entry sensors	Infrared sensor records entry to facility and sensor in soap dispenser records soap use.	London School of Hygiene and Tropical Medicine	2009	London	Judah, G., R. Aunger, W. P. Schmidt, S. Michie, S. Granger, and V. Curtis. 2009. "Experimental Pretesting of Hand-Washing Interventions in a Natural Setting." *American Journal of Public Health* 99 (Suppl 2): S405–11. https://www.ncbi.nlm.nih.gov/pubmed/19797755

Note: DfID = U.K. Department for International Development; GPS = Global Positioning System; GSM = Global System for Mobile Communications; ICT = information and communication technology; JMP = Joint Monitoring Programme; NGO = nongovernmental organization; RFID = radiofrequency identification; SIM = subscriber identification module; SMS = Short Message Service; UNESCO = United Nations Educational, Scientific, and Cultural Organization; UNICEF = United Nations Children's Fund; USAID = U.S. Agency for International Development; WASH = water, sanitation, and hygiene; WSP = Water and Sanitation Program.

www.ingramcontent.com/pod-product-compliance
Lightning Source LLC
Chambersburg PA
CBHW080426270326
41929CB00018B/3180